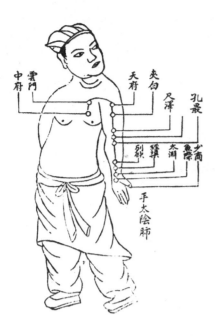

Chinese Medicine Workbook
A Comprehensive Review in 10 Weeks

- Theory & Diagnosis
- Channel Pathways
- Acupuncture
- Single Herbs
- Formulas
- Internal Medicine

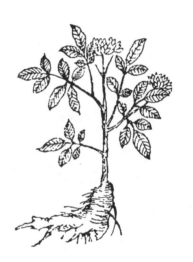

Jasmine Rose Oberste, L.Ac., M.S.TCM

THREE TREASURES PUBLISHING

San Francisco

THREE TREASURES PUBLISHING

94 29th Street
San Francisco, CA 94131
www.threetreasurespublishing.com

Cover images: Bai Zhi (*Angelica dahurica*) from Li Shizhen's *Bencao Gangmu* and Pericardium channel

Oberste, Jasmine R.
          Chinese Medicine Workbook : A Comprehensive Review in 10 Weeks

ISBN-13: 978-1973705314
ISBN-10: 1973705311

1. Chinese Medicine   2. Acupuncture   3. TCM   4. Chinese Herbal Medicine

Printed in the United States of America

To my teachers and students,
who, together, constitute the beautiful stream that is lineage medicine.

I am deeply grateful for what I've learned from all of you.

My mentor Dr. Robert Johns' teacher Dr. Andrew E. Tseng said,

"You can study medical texts for ten years
and find no such patients in the clinic.

You can work in the clinic for ten years and
find no such patients in any medical book."

This workbook is intended to support students in their initial endeavor of studying Chinese Medicine. From here we hope that you connect deeply with one or more of the living lineage traditions of Chinese Medicine that are at once more complex and simpler than any text could teach.

Chinese Medicine Workbook:
A Comprehensive Review in 10 Weeks

CONTENTS

Note: This workbook may be used for first or second year students: for students at the end of their first year, skip the formulas section at the end of each chapter and work through the rest of the material.

How to use this workbook

We encourage you to work with one or two other students at a regularly scheduled meeting time each week. Using your source texts (outlined below), look up the answers for each section.

SOURCE TEXTS:

- Channel Pathway Descriptions, Ear Point Illustration and Scalp Chart:
  Bensky, Dan *Acupuncture A Comprehensive Text*
  Shanghai College of Traditional Medicine Hardcover, 1996.

- Acupuncture Point Location & Indications, Channel Illustrations, Theory & Diagnosis:
  Xinnong, Cheng. *Chinese Acupuncture and Moxibustion*
  Foreign Languages Press; 3rd Edition 2009

- Theory & Diagnosis:
  Maciocia, Giovanni. *The Foundations of Chinese Medicine: A Comprehensive Text,*
  Churchill Livingstone; 3 edition 2015.

- Single Herbs:
  Bensky, Dan. *Chinese Herbal Medicine: Materia Medica*
  Eastland Press; 3 edition 2015

- Herbal Formulas:
  Scheid, Volker et al *Chinese Herbal Medicine: Formulas & Strategies*
  Eastland Press; 2nd edition 2015

    Additional recommended reading for studying Herbs:

    Yang, Yifan *Chinese Herbal Medicines: Comparisons and Characteristics*
    Churchill Livingstone; 2 edition 2010

    Zeng, Dafang *Essentials of Chinese Medicine : Materia Medica*
    Bridge Pub. Group 2003

How do we learn?

- *Engaging the different senses when studying* helps deepen our ability to remember new things: visual, listening, movement, speaking (not only reading). Try taking a walk with flashcards.

- *Preview, Study & Review*
    1. review last week's material
    2. study the current week's material in-depth
    3. preview (quick overview) of next week's material

*Times of exam preparation are an excellent time to practice what we learn
about the impacts of lifestyle (both positive & negative) on our health.*

Health in Chinese medicine may be defined as the **UNINHIBITED FLOW OF QI** 氣
Following are some thoughts on how we nourish our Qi and Blood and support their free flow

Post-Natal Qi is replenished from:
EATING :: BREATHING :: SLEEPING

Eating:
- Warm food, easy for Spleen to digest (especially in Fall & Winter)
- Eat & only eat (no studying, working, t.v.)
- Don't eat too fast or too much
- When you're hungry, stop & eat food (not caffeine)
- Eat breakfast (Stomach time: 7-9am)
- Eat dinner by around 6pm (not too late)

Breathing:
- Move your body regularly & gently (taiji, qigong, restorative walks…)
  (Health is demonstrated by a smooth flow of Qi & Blood)
- Consider a daily meditation or mindfulness practice

Sleeping:
- Take an afternoon nap. If you don't fall sleep, close your eyes & relax .
- Be asleep by 11pm
  (the GB & Liver recover their energy passively by resting at this time)
- Allow yourself enough time to sleep (aim for 8-9 hours)

In addition to the above, remember that **the body** thrives on rhythm & **regularity:**
- Eat & Sleep at regular times
- Schedule treatments for the whole quarter or semester leading up to your exams
  (acupuncture, body work, herbs…)
- Set up a study schedule, preferably with one or two other students and follow it

Acupuncture Overview

	Lu	LI	St	Sp	Ht	SI	UB	K	Pc	SJ	GB	Liv
Xi-Cleft												
Luo												
Yuan-Source												
Front Mu												
Back Shu												
Jing-Well												
Ying-Spring												
Shu-Stream												
Jing-River												
He-Sea												
Lower He-Sea												

8 Influential Points

Zang	
Fu	
Qi	
Blood	
Sinews	
Marrow	
Bones	
Vessels	

Eight Extra Meridians

	Confluent	Paired	Xi Cleft	Luo
Ren				
Du				
Dai				
Chong				
Yin Qiao				
Yang Qiao				
Yin Wei				
Yang Wei				

We recommend that students can fill out this chart completely in less than 5 minutes.

At the start of any major exam (comprehensive, board licensing, etc) write out the whole chart to use as a reference during your exam.

Lung- *Hand Tai Yin*

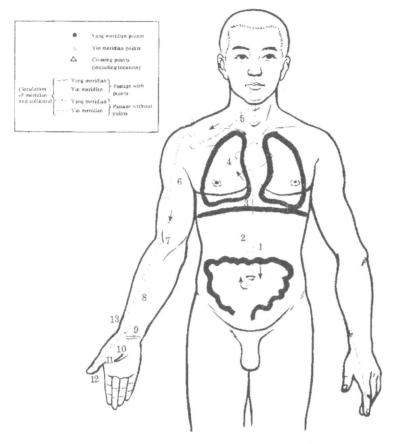

Fig. 5. The Lung Meridian of Hand-Taiyin

Originates:

Connects with
   Organs:
   Structures:

Xi:
Luo:
Yuan:

Front *Mu*:
Back *Shu*:

Jing Well:
Ying Spring:
Shu Stream:
Jing River:
He Sea

Influential Point (tissue):

Confluent Point (8 extras):
of which channel:

Command Point (area):

Crossing Points: none

Channel Pathway

This channel begins in the region of the **Stomach** (the so-called **middle burner**) and passes downward to connect with the **Large Intestine**. Returning, it follows the **cardiac orifice,** crosses the **diaphragm,** and **enters its associated Organ, the Lung**. Emerging transversely from the area between the Lung and **the throat**, the channel descends along the anterior aspect of the upper arm, lateral to the Heart and Pericardium channels. Reaching the elbow, it continues along the anterior aspect of the forearm to the anterior margin of the styloid process at the wrist. From here, it crosses the **radial artery** at the pulse, and extends over the thenar eminence to the radial side of the tip of the thumb.

A **branch** splits from the main channel above the styloid process at the wrist (Lu 7) and travels directly to the radial side of the tip of the index finger (LI 1)

This channel is associated with the Lung and connects with the Large Intestine.

Lung Channel Sx: fever and sensitivity to cold, nasal congestion, headache, pain in the chest, clavicle, shoulder and back, chills and pain along the channel on the arm

Lung Organ Sx: coughing, asthma, shortness of breath, fullness in the chest, parched throat, changes in the color of urine, irritability, blood in the sputum, palms hot; sometimes accompanied by distended abdomen and loose stool.

*Image from CAM, description from ACT

Large Intestine- Hand Yang Ming

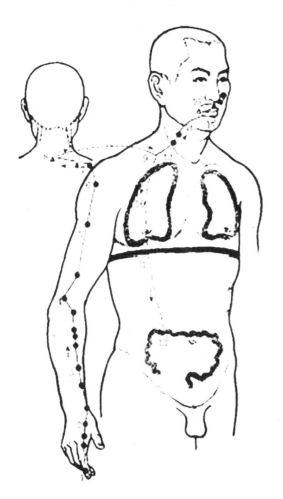

Originates:

Connects with
    Organs:
    Structures:

Xi:
Luo:
Yuan:

Front *Mu*:
Back *Shu:*

Jing Well:
Ying Spring:
Shu Stream:
Jing River:
He Sea
Lower *He* Sea:

Command Point (area):

Crossing Pts:

Channel Pathway

    This channel begins at the radial side of the tip of the index finger (LI 1) and proceeds upward between the first and second metacarpal bones of the hand. It then passes between the tendons of the *extensor pollicis longus* and *brevis* at the wrist and continues along the radial margin of the forearm to the lateral side of the elbow. From here it rises along the lateral aspect of the upper arm to the shoulder joint, then crosses behind the shoulder following the anterior margin of the acromion before turning upward. Just beneath the spinous process of the 7th cervical vertebra **(Du 14),** the channel enters directly into the **supraclavicular fossa**, and connects with the **Lung** before descending across the **diaphragm** to the **Large Intestine.**

    A **branch** separates from the main channel at the **supraclavicular fossa** and moves upward through the neck, crosses the cheek and enters the **lower gum**. From here, it curves around the lip (Du 26) and intersects the same channel coming from the opposite side of the body at the **philtrum**. The branch finally terminates at the side of the nose.

    According to chapter 4 of the *Ling Shu*, another **branch** descends to St 37 (*Shang Ju Xu*), the Lower He Sea point of the Large Intestine.

    This channel is associated with the Large Intestine and connects with the Lung

Large Intestine Channel Sx: fever, parched mouth and thirst, sore throat, nosebleed, toothache, red and painful eyes, swelling of the neck, pain along the course of the channel on the upper arm, shoulder and shoulder blade, motor impairment of the fingers

Large Intestine Organ Sx: abdominal pain, intestinal noises, loose stool; sometimes accompanied by shortness of breath and belching.

*Image from CAM, description from ACT

LUNG SYNDROMES

	Tongue	Pulse	Cough	Phlegm	Thirst	Sweating	HA	SOB	Other Sx.
Lung Qi Def									
Lung Yin Def									
Lung Wind Cold									
Lung Wind Heat									
Lung Phlegm Damp									
Lung Phlegm Heat									

LARGE INTESTINE SYNDROMES

	Tongue	Pulse	Sx
LI Damp Heat			
LI Dryness			

Five *Shu* Points

ZANG FU	*Jing* Well	*Ying* Spring	*Shu* Stream	*Jing* River	*He* Sea	Lower *He* Sea
Lung						x
Large Intestine						
Stomach						x
Spleen						x
Heart						x
Small Intestine						
Urinary Bladder						x
Kidney						x
Pericardium						x
San Jiao						
Gallbladder						x
Liver						x

Yin Channels start with which element:
Yang Channels start with which element:

 Shen Disturbance (Mental/Spirit problems):
Febrile Conditions:
Stifling/Distension in Chest:
Cough, Asthma/Wheezing with Fever:
Wind Damp Joint Pain:
Fu Organs:
Emergency Revival/Restore Consciousness:
Muscle/Channel Problems:
Change in Complexion:
Change in Voice:

Wood
木

_____   _____

_____   _____

Theory & Diagnosis
陰 陽
Yin and Yang

The earliest known text to make reference to Yin and Yang is the *Yi Jing* (or *I Ching* 易經, Book of Changes) in which Yin & Yang are symbolized by: _____ & ___ ___

Which of the following are Yin within Yin, Yang within Yin etc.
Yearly Cycle	Daily Cycle
Summer:	Dawn to Noon:
Autumn:	Noon to Dusk:
Winter:	Dusk to Midnight:
Spring:	Midnight to Dawn:

The five aspects of Yin Yang relationship are:
1.
2.
3.
4.
5.

These five aspects are illustrated in the *Tai Ji* (Yin Yang) symbol:

五行
Five Phases / Elements

TABLE OF FIVE PHASES CORRESPONDENCES

	木 WOOD	火 FIRE	土 EARTH	金 METAL	水 WATER
Direction					
Climatic Condition					
Season					
Process					
Color					
Taste					
Smell					
Yin Organ (Zang)					
Yang Organ (Fu)					
Opening					
Tissue					
Emotion					
Manifests in					
Human Sound					

The Four Diagnostic Methods: Intro

1. Looking (Inspection)
(Tongue portion of "Looking" will be week 6)

Complexion / Face Color:
Red:
>   Whole Face:
>   Malar Flush:

White/Pale:
>   Bright white, puffy:
>   Withered, pale:
Yellow:
>   Face Pale Yellow without Brightness:
>   Face & Body Bright Orange:
>   Face & Body Smoky Dark Yellow:
Blue/Green:
Grey or Blackish:
(CAM says grey, Maciocia says black):

Secretions (nasal, sputum, urine, vaginal discharge)
Clear or white:
Turbid, yellow:

2. Listening & Smelling (Auscultation and Olfaction)
Listening:
Voice
>   Sudden Loss:
>   Gradual Loss:
>   Loud, Coarse:
>   Weak, Thin:
>   Reluctant to Talk:
>   Incessant Talking:
>   (also see "5 Phase" chart, human sound)
>   Soliliquoy:

Breathing
>   Course, Loud: vs.   Weak, Thin:

Cough:
>   Loud, Explosive: vs.   Weak:
>   Dry:

Smelling (according to 5 Phases/Elements)
Rancid: Sweet: Putrid:
Burnt: Rank:

Strong, Foul Smell:
Absence of Smell:
Bad Breath:

3. Asking (Inquiry)   **4. Feeling (Palpation)**
10 Questions: week 7   Pulse: week 5

week 1

WARM, ACRID, RELEASE THE EXTERIOR

herb (yao 藥)	flavor (wei 味)		temp (qi 氣)	channels				
ma huang	**acrid**, sl. bitter		**warm**	**Lu**	**UB**			
gui zhi	**acrid**, sweet		**warm**	**Lu**	**UB**	Ht		
zi su ye	**acrid**	aromatic	**warm**	**Lu**		Sp		
jing jie	**acrid**	aromatic	sl. warm	**Lu**			Liv	
fang feng	**acrid**, sweet		sl. warm		**UB**	Sp	Liv	
qiang huo	**acrid**, bitter	aromatic	**warm**		**UB**			Kid
gao ben	**acrid**		**warm**		**UB**			
bai zhi	**acrid**		**warm**	**Lu**			St	
xi xin	**acrid**		**warm**	**Lu**				Kid
sheng jiang	**acrid**		**warm**	**Lu**		Sp	St	
cong bai	**acrid**		**warm**	**Lu**			St	
xiang ru	**acrid**	aromatic	sl. warm	**Lu**			St	
xin yi hua	**acrid**		**warm**	**Lu**			St	

COOL, ACRID, RELEASE THE EXTERIOR

herb (yao 藥)	flavor (wei 味)		temp (qi 氣)	channels							
bo he	**acrid**	aromatic	**cooling**	**Lu**	**Liv**						
niu bang zi	**acrid**, bitter		**cold**	**Lu**			St				
chan tui	sweet, salty		**sl. cold**	**Lu**	**Liv**						
sang ye	sweet, bitter		**cold**	**Lu**	**Liv**						
ju hua	sweet, bitter		**sl. cold**	**Lu**	**Liv**						
man jing zi	bitter, **acrid**		**cool**		**Liv**		St				
dan dou chi	sweet, sl bitter		**cold** or warm	**Lu**			St				
fu ping	**acrid**		**cold**	**Lu**						UB	
mu zei	sweet, bitter		**neutral**	**Lu**	**Liv**						
ge gen	sweet, **acrid**		**cool**				St	Sp			
chai hu	bitter, **acrid**		**cool**		**Liv**	GB			SJ/Pc		
sheng ma	sweet, **acrid**		**cool**	**Lu**			St	Sp			LI

CLEAR HEAT, PURGE FIRE

herb (yao 藥)	flavor (wei 味)	temp (qi 氣)	channels									
shi gao	sweet, acrid	**very cold**	Lu	**St**								
zhi mu	**bitter**	**cold**	Lu	**St**	K							
zhi zi	**bitter**	**cold**	Lu	**St**		Liv	SJ					
dan zhu ye	sweet, bland	**cold**		**St**				SI	Ht			
xia ku cao	**bitter**, acrid	**cold**				Liv				GB		
lian xin	**bitter**	**cold**							Ht		Pc	
lu gen	sweet	**cold**	Lu	**St**								
jue ming zi	**bitter**, sweet	**cool**			K	Liv						LI
mi meng hua	sweet	**cool**				Liv						
gu jing cao	sweet	neutral		**St**		Liv						

Herbs

Warm, Acrid, Release the Exterior

Ma Huang	*Fang Feng*	*Xi Xin*	*Xin Yi Hua*
Gui Zhi	*Qiang Huo*	*Sheng Jiang*	*(Cang Er Zi)*
Zi Su Ye	*Gao Ben*	*Cong Bai*	
Jing Jie	*Bai Zhi*	*Xiang Ru*	

1. _____ , _____, _____ & _____ are good for treating **nasal congestion**.

2. _____ is best for ***Jue Yin* vertex headache**. (Enters the UB channel only)

3. _____ is best for ***Yang Ming* frontal headache**. (Enters the *Yang Ming* Stomach channel, and Lung channel)

4. _____ is best for ***Tai Yang* occipital headache**. Additionally it guides to the *Tai Yang* and Du channels. (Enters the *Tai Yang* UB channel and Kidney channel)

5. _____ is best for ***Shao Yin* headache**. Some traditional texts put this herb in "Warm the Interior" category, emphasizing its functions of entering the Kidney (*Shao Yin*) channel to warm the interior and disperse cold.

The only two herbs from this category that **enter the Liver channel** are often used together to **expel Wind.**
6. _____ can be used for either Wind-Cold or Wind-Heat. In its charred form it is used to stop bleeding.
7. _____ can be used for either External Wind or Internal Wind. It also treats Wind Cold Damp.

8. In addition to relieving Wind Cold, _____ also moves qi to treat **morning sickness** and **calm a restless fetus**.

9. **Caution** not to use more than 1 qian (3 grams) of _____ .

10. _____ is the only herb in this category that **enters the Heart channel**. It warms and facilitates the flow of Yang Qi in the chest (for palpitations). Also harmonizes the *Ying* and *Wei* (with Bai Shao)

11. _____ is used for **exterior Excess Cold** conditions, is effective in opening the pores, controls wheezing, and promotes urination to treat edema.

12. _____, mild in its exterior releasing function, is regarded as the **imperial anti-emetic** herb to treat all patterns of vomiting, especially due to rebellious Stomach Qi with Stomach Cold. Additionally it harmonizes the *Ying* and *Wei* (with Hong Zao).

Cool, Acrid, Release the Exterior

Bo He	*Sang Ye*	*Dan Dou Chi*	*Ge Gen*
Niu Bang Zi	*Ju Hua*	*Fu Ping*	*Chai Hu*
Chan Tui	*Man Jing Zi*	*Mu Zei*	*Sheng Ma*

1. _____ **treats irritability** and can be warm or cool depending on its preparation.

These three herbs all release the exterior and **raise sunken Yang Qi**.

2. _____ is most famous for treating ***Shao Yang*** stage disorder (including malaria) and therefore enters both *Shao Yang* channels (GB & SJ) and their *biao-li* associated channels (Liver & Pericardium).

3. _____ vents rashes, **guides other herbs upward**, and treats fire toxin especially in the upper or superficial part of the body. (Lung & LI. channels to treat the skin with acupuncture. Also enters Stomach & Spleen)

4. _____, mildest in its Yang raising function, **releases the muscle layer** to treat stiff neck and upper back and nourishes fluids. Its Yang raising function addresses diarrhea (therefore entering the Spleen channel).

Many of the herbs in this category treat **sore throat**.

5. _____ is especially good for **loss of voice** and spasms.

6. _____ is especially good for **cough** from Lung Heat or Lung Dryness.

7. _____ specifically benefits the throat, and also lubricates the intestines.

8. _____ treats sore throat from fire toxin.

Many of the herbs in this category **treat the eyes**, and they all enter the Liver channel*.

9. _____ also **spreads constrained Liver qi**.

10. _____ is sweet to nourish the Liver and Kidney, for Liver/Kidney yin deficiency or Liver Yang rising.

11. _____ is also bitter to drain Heat from the Lung, and treats Lung Dryness.

12. _____ & Chan Tui both **clear visual obstruction**.

13. Herbs that **promote the expression of rashes:**
_____, _____, _____, _____, & _____ (also Fu Ping).

14. Use _____ with **caution during pregnancy**
    (*any animal / insect products generally caution or C/I in pregnancy)

Clear Heat, Drain Fire

Shi Gao   Dan Zhu Ye   Jue Ming Zi   Gu Jing Cao
Zhi Mu   Xia Ku Cao   Qing Xiang Zi   Tian Hua Fen (Phlegm Heat)
Zhi Zi   Lu Gen   Mi Meng Hua

1. _____ , bitter and cold, is the only herb in this category that **enriches yin and moistens dryness.**

2. _____ & _____ , the only two herbs in this category that enter the Heart channel, **treat irritability**.

3. The five herbs in this category that **treat the eyes** all enter the Liver channel (for such things as red, painful, swollen eyes, superficial visual obstruction, and spots in front of the eyes)
_____ , _____ , _____ , _____ & _____

4. _____ , the only herb in this category that enters the Large Intestine channel, **moistens the intestine & unblocks the bowel.**

5. _____ , enters the Liver & GB, and **dissipates nodules.**

6. _____ , _____ , & _____ all clear **Qi Level Heat** from the Lung and Stomach. Of these, which is strongest?

7. _____ , the only herb in this category that enters the San Jiao channel, **eliminates Damp Heat** for painful urinary dysfunction and jaundice.

8. _____ & _____ are both sweet and cold, and they **promote urination.** Of these two, which one **generates fluids**?

9. Two herbs in this category enter the Kidney channel.
_____ enriches Kidney yin, for Kidney Yin deficiency, and
_____ for Liver Yin Def causing constipation or Liver Yang rising affecting the eyes.

10. **Contraindicated in pregnancy,** _____ drains Lung Heat, transforms phlegm, and **generates fluids.**

DUI YAO
Synergistic Herb Combinations

<u>Ma Huang & Xing Ren</u>
Both enter the Lung channel.
One is acrid to disperse and open.
The other is bitter to descend and drain.
Together they restore the function of Lung Qi
to **stop coughing and wheezing**.
    Ma Huang Tang
    Ge Gen Tang
    Ma Xing Shi Gan Tang

<u>Bai Shao & Gui Zhi</u>
One is cool, sour and astringent, assisting the yin.
The other is warm, acrid and dispersing, assisting the yang.
Together they drain without damaging the yin, and constrain yin without retaining pathogens.
In combination they **harmonize the *ying* and *wei***.
    Gui Zhi Tang
    Ge Gen Tang (Gui Zhi Tang plus: Ma Huang, Ge Gen)
    Xiao Jian Zhong Tang (Gui Zhi Tang plus: Yi Tang)

<u>Da Zao & Sheng Jiang</u> (good for morning sickness)
Da Zao moderates the pungent, moving nature of Sheng Jiang
Sheng Jiang balances out the accumulative effects of Da Zao.
One tonifies, acting on the *ying*.
The other moves, acting on the *wei*.
Together they support the *zheng qi*, expel pathogen, and **harmonize the *ying* and *wei***.
    (milder than *Bai Shao & Gui Zhi*)

<u>Jie Geng & Xing Ren</u>
One guides up and diffuses.
The other descends and drains.
Together they regulate the Lung's function of diffusing and descending Qi
to transform and disperse phlegm, **stop cough and calm wheezing**.
    Sang Ju Yin

<u>Ma Huang & Gui Zhi</u>
Ma Huang strongly opens the pores, while Gui Zhi pushes out the pathogen.
Together they mutually reinforce each other
Together they are very effective in **promoting perspiration
and releasing excess exterior wind cold** (especially the muscle layer).
    Ma Huang Tang
    Ge Gen Tang
    Xiao Qing Long Tang

Formulas:
Release Exterior

Ma Huang Tang   **Sang Ju Yin**   *Xin Yi San*
Gui Zhi Tang   **Yin Qiao San**   **Ge Gen Tang**
Xiao Qing Long Tang   **Chai Ge Jie Ji Tang**   **Ren Shen Bai Du San**
Jiu Wei Qiang Huo Tang   *Chuan Xiong Cha Tiao San*

(State Board Formulas in **bold**)

External Wind
1. Wind with Headache:

Wind Cold
2. Excess W/C with wheezing:
3. Excess W/C in muscle layer with stiff neck/upper back:
4. W/C in muscle layer, with *ying/wei* disharmony:
5. W/C with nasal congestion:
6. W/C with fluid in Lungs:

Wind Cold Damp (with Deficiency)
7. W/C/D with Qi deficiency:

Wind Cold with Internal Heat
8. Ext W/C in muscle layer transforming into heat:
    (the above formula is *Tai Yang- Yang Ming* combination disease)
9. W/C/Damp with Internal Heat:

Wind Heat
10. W/H with Cough:
11. Wind Heat with Heat Toxin:

Ma Huang Tang   *Gui Zhi Tang*   *Ge Gen Tang*
1.   1.   =Gui Zhi Tang plus:
2.   2.   1.
3.   plus 3 amigos   2.
4.

	Sang Ju Yin	Yin Qiao San
	Jie Geng, Lian Qiao, Bo He, Gan Cao, Lu Gen	
Herbs:	Sang Ye, Ju Hua, Xing Ren	Jin Yin Hua, Niu Bang Zi, Jing Jie, Dan Dou Chi, Dan Zhu Ye
Fxn:	Promotes sweating, releases Exterior Wind-Heat	
Emphasis:	Disperses Lung Qi	Clears Heat Toxin
Sx (common):	Fever & chills, thirst, headache, sore throat	
	T: think yellow coat P: floating, rapid	
Sx (different):	cough	boils, sores

Meridians & Points

Stomach- Foot Yang Ming

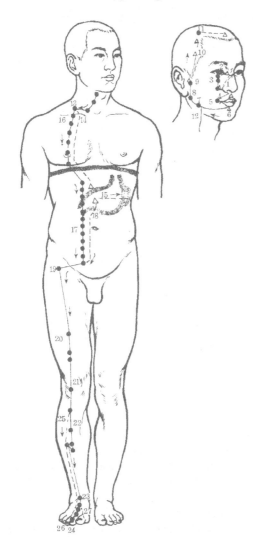

Fig. 7 The Stomach Meridian of Foot-Yangming

Originates:

Connects with
  Organs:
  Structures:

Xi:	*Jing* Well:
Luo:	*Ying* Spring:
Yuan:	*Shu* Stream:
	Jing River:
Front *Mu:*	*He* Sea
Back *Shu:*	

Large Intestine lower *He* Sea:
Small Intestine lower *He* Sea:

Large Intestine Front *Mu:*

Crossing Points:

Channel Pathway

This channel begins beside the nose (**LI 20**) then ascends of the root of the nose (**UB 1**) where it intersects with the Bladder channel. Descending along the lateral side of the nose, it enters the **upper gum** and joins the Governing channel at the **philtrum** (**Du 26**) then circles back around the corner of the mouth, meeting the Conception channel at the **mental labial groove** (**Ren 24**) on the chin. From here, it follows the angle of the jaw and runs upward in front of the ear. It proceeds along the hairline until it intersects the Gall Bladder channel at GB 6. Finally it crosses the middle of the forehead, parallel with the hairline, where it joins the Governing channel (**Du 24**)

One **branch (1)** separates from the main channel on the lower jaw and descends along the throat, entering the **supraclavicular fossa**. Here, it travels posteriorly to the upper back, where it meets the Governing channel at **Du 14** (*Da Zhui*). It proceed downward across the **diaphragm**, intersecting the Conception channel internally at points **Ren 13** (*Shangwan*) and **Ren 12** (*Zhongwan*) before entering its associated Organ, the **Stomach,** and communicating with the **Spleen.**

Another vertical **branch (2)** descends directly from the supraclavicular fossa along the mammillary line, then passes beside the umbilicus and through the lower abdomen to the inguinal region.

Yet another **branch (3)** begins at the **pylorus** and descends internally to the inguinal region where it joins with the vertical branch just described. From here, the channel crosses to point St 31 (*Biguan*) on the anterior aspect of the thigh, and descends directly to the patella. It then proceeds along the lateral side of the tibia to the dorsum of the foot, terminating at the lateral side of the tip of the second toe.

A parallel **branch (4)** separates from the main channel at St 36 (*Zusanli*), three units below the knee, and terminates at the lateral side of the middle toe.

Another **branch (5)** separates on the dorsum of the foot, at point St 42 (*Chongyang*) and terminates at the medial side of the big toe, where it connects with the Spleen channel at **Sp 1** (*Yinbai*)

Stomach Channel Sx: high fever, tidal fevers, flushed face, sweating and delirium, sometimes sensitivity to cold, or pain in the eyes, dry nostrils and nosebleed, fever blisters, sore throat, swelling on the neck, facial paralysis (mouth awry), chest pain, pain or distension along the course of the channel in the leg and foot, coldness in the lower limb.

Stomach Organ Sx: abdominal distension, fullness or edema, discomfort when reclining, seizures, persistent hunger, yellow urine.

*Image from CAM, description from ACT

Spleen- Foot Tai Yin

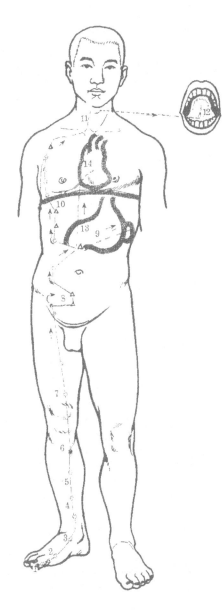

Fig. 8 The Spleen Meridian of Foot-Taiyin

Originates:

Connects with
 Organs:
 Structures:

Xi:
Luo:
Yuan:

Front *Mu*:
Back *Shu:*

Jing Well:
Ying Spring:
Shu Stream:
Jing River:
He Sea

Confluent point (8 extras):
Which channel:

Crossing Pts:

<u>Channel Pathway</u>

This channel begins on the medial tip of the big toe. From here, it follows the border between the dark and light skin of the medial aspect of the foot. It then passes in front of the medial malleolus and up the leg, along the posterior side of the tibia, crossing, and then traveling anterior to, the Liver channel. From here, it crosses over the medial aspect of the thigh and into the abdomen. There, after crossing the Conception channel at points **Ren 3** (*Zhongji*) and **Ren 4** (*Guanyuan*), the channel enters its associated Organ, the **Spleen**, and communicates with the **Stomach**. It then ascends across the **diaphragn** and intersects the Gall Bladder at point **GB 24** (*Riyue*), and the Liver channel at point **Liv 14** (*Qimen*). Continuing upward beside the **esophagus,** it crosses the Lung channel at point **Lu 1** (*Zhongfu*) and finally reaches the **root of the tongue**, dispersing over its lower surface.

A **branch** of this channel separates in the Stomach region and advances upward across the diaphragm, transporting Qi into the **Heart**.

Spleen Channel Sx: heaviness in the body or head, general feverishness, fatigued limbs and emaciated muscles, stiffness of the tongue, coldness along the medial side of the leg and knee, edema in the foot or leg.

Spleen Organ Sx: abdominal pain, fullness or distension, diarrhea, incomplete digestion of food, intestinal noises, vomiting, hard lumps in the abdomen, reduced appetite, jaundice, constipation.

*Image from CAM, description from ACT

SPLEEN SYNDROMES

	Tongue	Pulse	Complexion	Appetite	Stool	Dislike Speaking	Lassitude	Heaviness	Other Sx.
Spleen Qi Def									
Spleen Yang Def									
Spleen Damp Cold									
Spleen Damp Heat									
Spleen Not Controlling Blood									

STOMACH SYNDROMES

	Tongue	Pulse	Epigastrium	Reflux	Vomit	Hunger	Bowel	Other Sx.
Stomach Yin Def								
Cold Fluid Retention								
Food Retention								
Stomach Fire								

Jing **Well**

Indications: 1.
2.
3.

Lu___   St___   Ht___   UB___   P____   GB____
LI___   Sp___   SI___   K____   SJ____   Liv____

1. **Hernia,** enuresis, **uterine bleeding,** prolapse of uterus, epilepsy:
(direct moxa to treat uterine bleeding)

2. Abdominal distension, bloody stools, menorrhagia, **uterine bleeding**, mental disorders, dream disturbed sleep, convulsion:
(direct moxa for uterine bleeding together with Liv 1, or Liv 1 alone)

3. Facial swelling, **deviation of mouth**, epistaxis, toothache, sore throat and hoarse voice, abdominal distension, coldness in the leg and foot, febrile disease, dream disturbed sleep, mania:

4. Headache, nasal obstruction, epistaxis, opthalmalgia, **malposition of fetus**, difficult labor, detention of after birth, feverish sensation of sole:
(direct moxa to turn fetus)

5. Headache, redness of the eyes, sore throat, stiffness of the tongue, febrile disease, irritability:

6. Toothache, sore throat, swelling of the submandibular region, numbness of fingers, febrile disease with anhidrosis, loss of consciousness:

7. **Sore throat,** cough, asthma, epistaxis, fever, loss of consciousness, mania, spasmodic pain of the thumb:

8. Headache, febrile disease, loss of consciousness, **insufficient lactation**, sore throat, redness of the eye, **cloudiness of the cornea**:

9. **Migraine, deafness, tinnitus,** opthalmalgia, dream-disturbed sleep, febrile disease:

10. Headache, blurring of vision, dizziness, sore throat, dryness of the tongue, loss of voice, dysuria, **infantile convulsions**, feverish sensation in the sole, **loss of consciousness**:

11. Cardiac pain, palpitation, loss of consciousness, aphasia with stiffness & swelling of the tongue, febrile disease, heat stroke, convulsion, feverish palms:

12. Palpitation, cardiac pain, pain in the chest and hypochondriac region, mania, febrile disease, loss of consciousness:

Ying **Spring**

Indications: 1.

                 2.

                 3.

Lu___   St___   Ht___   UB___   P____   GB____

LI___   Sp___   SI___   K____   SJ___   Liv____

1. Cough, hemoptysis, **sore throat**, loss of voice, fever, feverish palms:

2. Pruritus vulvae, prolapse of uterus, irregular menstruation, nocturnal emission, hemoptysis, thirst, diarrhea, swelling and pain of the dorsum of the foot, acute infantile omphalitis*:
    (mild indirect moxa for Yin deficient Heat)

*omphalitis: inflammation of the umbilicus

3. Toothache, facial pain, **deviation of the mouth,** sore throat, epistaxis, gastric pain, acid regurgitation, abdominal distension, diarrhea, dysentery, constipation, swelling and pain of the dorsum of the foot, febrile disease:

4. Blurring vision, **epistaxis, toothache, sore throat**, febrile disease:

5. Abdominal distension, gastric pain, constipation, febrile disease with anhidrosis:

6. Headache, neck rigidity, blurring of vision, epistaxis, mania:

7. Numbness of the fingers, febrile disease, tinnitus, headache, reddish urine:

8. Palpitation, pain in the chest, spasmodic pain of the little finger, **feverish palms**, enuresis, **dysuria,** pruritus of the external genitalia:

9. **Cardiac pain, mental disorder**, epilepsy, gastritis, foul breath, **fungus infection of the hand and foot, vomiting, nausea:**

10. Headache, redness of the eyes, sudden deafness, sore throat, **malaria**, pain in the arm:

11. Headache, dizziness and vertigo, pain in the outer canthus, **tinnitus, deafness**, swelling of the cheek, **pain in the hypochondriac region**, distending pain of the breast, febrile disease:

12. **Pain in the hypochondrium**, abdominal distension, headache, dizziness, vertigo, congestion, swelling and pain of the eye, **deviation of the mouth, hernia**, painful urination, retention of urine, irregular menstruation, epilepsy, insomnia, convulsion:

Zang Fu

Governs Blood:

Stores Blood:

Governs Qi :

Governs Food Qi:

Stores Essence :

Influences Body Fluids:

Manifests in the complexion:

Manifests in the nails:

Influence the Wei Qi:

Loathes Dampness:

Origin of fluids:

Separates fluids:

Control dispersing and descending:

Avenue for the *yuan* qi:

Controls sinews:

Control channels and vessels:

Controls blood vessels:

Governs the four limbs:

Control the two lower orifices:

Control skin and (body) hair:

Root of pre-heaven qi:

Root of post-heaven qi:

Governs birth, growth, reproduction and development:

Controls sweat:

Ensures the smooth flow of Qi:

Houses Thought :

Houses the Mind:

House the Corporeal Spirit (*po* 魄):

Opens into the eyes:

Opens into the tongue:

Governs transformation and transportation:

Controls "rotting & ripening" of food:

Source of fire for all the internal organs:

Controls speech:

Governs the voice:

Controls the reception/grasping of Qi:

Loathes Wind:

Controls the muscles and the four limbs:

Controls the descending of qi:

Controls the raising Qi:

Produces Marrow, fill the brain control the bones:

Stores and excretes bile:

Controls receiving and transforming:

Root of yuan qi:

Manifest in the head hair:

Opens into the nose:

Arises from the left side (tongue and pulse):

Opens into the ears:

Holds/controls the Blood:

Removes water by Qi transformation (Qi Hua):

The Qi of the Upper burner is like:

The Qi of the Middle Burner is like:

The Qi of the Lower Burner is like a:

CLEAR HEAT, COOL BLOOD

herb (yao 藥)	flavor (wei 味)	temp (qi 氣)	channels				
Xi Jiao	bitter, salty	**cold**	Ht	Liv	St		
Shui Niu Jiao	salty	**cold**					
Sheng Di Huang	sweet, bitter	**cold**	Ht	Liv		K	
Xuan Shen	salty, sweet, bitter	**cold**			St	K	Lu
Mu Dan Pi	acrid, bitter	**cool**	Ht	Liv		K	
Zi Cao	sweet	**cold**	Ht	Liv			
Di Gu Pi	sweet	**cold**		Liv		K	Lu
Bai Wei	bitter, salty	**cold**			St	K	Lu
Yin Chai Hu	sweet	**cool**		Liv	St		

CLEAR HEAT TOXIN

herb (yao 藥)	flavor (wei 味)		temp (qi 氣)	channels						
Jin Yin Hua	sweet		**cold**		Lu	St			LI	
Lian Qiao	bitter, sl. acrid		**cool**	Ht				Liv	GB	
Da Qing Ye	bitter		**very cold**	Ht	Lu	St				
Qing Dai	salty		**cold**		Lu	St	Liv			
Ban Lan Gen	bitter		**cold**	Ht	Lu	St				
Pu Gong Ying	bitter, sweet		**cold**			St	Liv			
Zi Hu Di Ding	acrid, bitter		**cold**	Ht			Liv			
Ye Ju Hua	bitter, acrid		**sl. cold**		Lu		Liv			
Bai Jiang Cao	acrid, bitter		**sl. cold**			St	Liv		LI	
Yu Xing Cao	acrid		**cool**		Lu				LI	
Chuan Xin Lian	bitter		**cold**		Lu	St			LI	SI
Bai Hua She She Cao	bitter, sweet		**cold**			St	Liv		LI	
Bai Tou Weng	bitter		**cold**			St	Liv		LI	
Ya Dan Zi	bitter	**toxic**	**cold**				Liv		LI	
Ma Chi Xian	sour		**cold**				Liv		LI	
Hong Teng	bitter		neutral				Liv		LI	
Bai Xian Pi	bitter		**cold**			St	Sp			
Tu Fu Ling	sweet, bland		neutral			St	Liv			
Ma Bo	acrid		neutral		Lu					
Shan Dou Gen	bitter		**cold**		Lu				LI	
She Gan	bitter		**cold**		Lu					
Lou Lu	bitter, salty		**cold**			St			LI	
Lu Dou	(clear summer heat)									
Qing Hao	(clear summer heat)									
Niu Huang	(open orifices)									
Chang Shan	(expel parasites)									

Herbs

Clear Heat, Cool Blood

Xi Jiao	*Xuan Shen*	*Di Gu Pi*	*Chi Shao* (Invigorate Blood)
Shui Niu Jiao	*Mu Dan Pi*	*Bai Wei*	
Sheng Di Huang	*Zi Cao*	*Yin Chai Hu*	

These three herbs all **clear Heat and cool Blood**, for heat lodged in the *ying* and blood level.

1. _____ is also **invigorates blood** and dispels stasis due to heat consuming fluid in the blood.

2. _____ is sweet, cold, moist and juicy to **nourish the yin**.

3. _____ is salty and cold to **soften hardness, relieve toxicity** (sore throat), and dissipate nodules for scrofula.

4. _____ & _____ are both salty and cold to **clear blood heat and relieve toxicity**, and are the primary herbs for **heat lodged in the nutritive and blood level** of Warm Febrile Disease (to treat high fever, loss of consciousness, convulsions and epilepsy and bleeding)

5. One of the few herbs that **moistens the intestines and unblocks** the bowel that is not a seed, _____ also clears blood heat and fire toxicity to **vent rashes**, and **clears damp-heat** from the skin.

6. Often put in the 'Invigorate Blood' category, _____ clears Liver Fire, injury and treats gynecological problems.

7. _____ enters the Lung, Liver and Kidney, drains **fire from yin deficiency**, clears Lung Heat and **stops coughing**, and drains floating fire in the kidney channel (toothache). Additionally, it is the root bark of a common blood tonic berry.

8. _____ treats **childhood nutritional impairment** with heat.

9. _____ promotes urination, cools blood and relieves toxicity.

Review Heat Sx:

Ying level Heat Sx:

Blood Level Heat Sx:

Clear Heat Toxin

Jin Yin Hua	Ziu Hua Di Ding	Ma Chi Xian	Lou Lu
Ren Dong Teng	Bai Jiang Cao	Hong Teng	Lu Dou (Summer Heat)
Lian Qiao	Yu Xing Cao	Bai Xian Pi (D/H)	Qing Hao (Summer Heat)
Da Qing Ye	Chuan Xin Lian	Tu Fu Ling	Niu Huang (Open Orifices)
Qing Dai	Bai Hua She She Cao	Ma Bo	Chang Shan (Expel Parasites)
Ban Lan Gen	Bai Tou Weng	Shan Dou Gen	
Pu Gong Ying	Ya Dan Zi	She Gan	

1. _____ **promotes lactation**, treats abscesses and nodules, and d/h causing jaundice or painful urination.

These two herbs, often used together, they release **exterior Wind Heat**.
2. _____ treats hot sores of the breast, throat, and eyes, or internal abscesses and clears Damp Heat in the lower burner.
3. _____ dissipates nodules.

Many herbs in this category treat **sore throat**.
4. Two for Wind Heat:_____ & _____
5. _____ enters only the Lung channel, and is sometimes used alone for sore throat, and it **strongly clears phlegm** from the Lungs.
6. _____ also enters only the Lung channel, and is good for **loss of voice** and cough due to Lung Heat.
7. _____ enters the Lung & L.I., also good for cough due to Lung Heat and d/h jaundice.
8. _____ (the leaf) cools blood for skin blotches & _____ (the root of the same plant) benefits the throat, cools blood, and treats Damp Heat jaundice.
9. _____ clears heat from the Lungs, throat, and urinary tract and also dries Dampness for Damp Heat dysentery, hot painful urination and eczema.   Very bitter!

These two "cao" herbs relieve toxicity and promote purulent discharge.
10. _____ is primarily for **Lung abscess**.
11. _____ is primarily for **intestinal abscess**.

12. In some parts of China _____ is used as a substitute for *Ji Xue Teng*. This herb invigorates blood to treat trauma, dysmenorrhea and joint pain, and treats toxic abscesses.

13. _____ clears heat, opens the orifices, awakens the *shen*, vaporizes phlegm, clears the Liver, extinguishes wind, and stops tremors.

Two herbs listed above clear Summer Heat.
14. _____ clears Summer Heat with thirst as a key Sx, and is an antidote to *Fu Zi.*
15. _____ treats deficient fever, malaria, and cools blood to stop bleeding.

16. _____ treats dysentery and is used topically for warts.

17. Use _____ with caution, as it induces vomiting to expel phlegm and is toxic. It treats malaria (Bensky puts it in the 'Expel Parasites' category)

Qing Hao, Di Gu Pi, and *Yin Chai Hu* all reduce yin deficient heat.
18. _____ relieves summer heat.
19. _____ clears Liver Heat.
20. _____ drains Lung Heat.

21. _____ clears Damp Heat by promoting urination, for hot painful urinary dysfunction and Damp Heat jaundice. In modern times used in anti-cancer formulas in large dose (1 liang or more), often in combination with Ban Zhi Lian.

22. _____ clears Damp Heat from the skin, for ulcers and other hot skin lesions. Also relieves toxicity and relives damp for painful urination or damp-heat jaundice.

Caution & Contra-Indicated During Pregnancy

Mu Dan Pi- C/I during pregnancy (or excess menstruation)
Ma Chi Xian- C/I during pregnancy
She Gan- C/I during pregnancy
Lou Lu- C/I during pregnancy

Xi Jiao- with great caution during pregnancy
Sheng Di-C/I in pregnant women with blood def. or Sp/St def.
Bai Hua She She Cao- caution during pregnancy
Ya Dan Zi- caution during pregnancy (and in children)
Hong Teng- caution during pregnancy
Qing Hao- C/I in post-partum women with blood def, or cold from Sp/St def.

Wen Bing
溫病

	Wei	*Qi*	*Ying*	*Xue*
Location	exterior	interior		
Common Sx:	fever, thirst, red tongue, rapid pulse			
Fever	fever	high fever	fever at night	
Chills	slight	none		
Thirst	slight	severe	mild	mild
Sweating	slight	profuse	possible night sweats	
Mental	none	restlessness	restlessness/delirium	delirium/coma
Skin	none	none	erythema/purpura	
Bleeding	no			yes
Tongue	normal or red tip	red body yellow coating	deep red	deep red with prickles
Pulse	rapid & floating	rapid & forceful	rapid & thin	

Four Stages (Wen Bing) Review Questions:
What Sx do all four stages have in common (including T & P):
Which stage is exterior:
Which one has bleeding:
Which one has a high fever:
Which one's tongue may be normal:
Which two have skin rash:
     Of these two, which one is darker & more severe:
Which one may have chills:

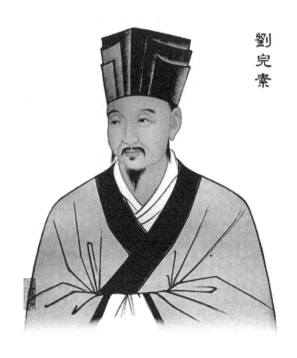

劉
完
素

Liu Wan-su (1120-1200) observed the high frequency of fever and inflammation in serious diseases and promoted the idea of using herbs of cooling nature to treat these conditions. This was a step in the opposite direction of many of his predecessors, who focused on using warming herbs. This work had much influence on the later concept of "wen bing" or epidemic febrile diseases, which corresponded to (and preceded) the Western concept of contageous disease. He also undertook a detailed study of the Nei Ching Su Wen [Nei Jing Su Wen], describing the etiology of disease in relation to the teachings of that famous text. (*www.itmonline.org*)

DUI YAO
Synergistic Herb Combinations

Shi Gao & Zhi Mu
One clears, the other moistens.
Together they strongly clear and drain deficient heat
While **protecting fluids and Yin**.
Together **they clear deficient Heat from the Lungs and Stomach.**
> *Bai Hu Tang*

Shi Gao & Zhu Ye
One is heavy, down bearing, and draining.
The other is light, upbearing, and dispelling.
Together they clear heat in the upper and lower body, the Interior and Exterior.
Together they **clear Heat in the Lungs, Stomach, and Heart,**
Eliminate vexation and **stop thirst**.
> *Zhu Ye Shi Gao Tang*

Ma Huang & Shi Gao
One is warm, diffuses, and scatters cold
The other is cold, down-bears and clears heat.
Together, they effectively **diffuse the lungs and calm asthma,**
Disinhibit urination and disperse swelling,
Clear heat and drain Fire.
> *Ma Xing Shi Gan Tang*

Jin Yin Hua & Lian Qiao
Both are light, clearing, floating, diffusing, and dissipating.
Together, they strongly and effectively **clear heat and resolve toxins.**
> *Yin Qiao San*
> *Qing Ying Tang*

Chai Hu & Huang Qin
One dispels external evils and raises clear Yang.
The other drains internal evils and downbears turbidity.
Together they **harmonize the *Shao Yang*,**
the Interior and the Exterior, and the Liver and Gall Bladder.
Together they eliminate Liver/Gall Bladder Damp Heat.
> *Long Dan Xie Gan Tang*
> *Pu Ji Xiao Du Yin*
> *Xiao Chai Hu Tang*

Huang Lian & Huang Qin
Together they **clear Heat, dry Damp,**
Drain Fire, and resolve toxins from the
Upper, middle, and lower burners.
> *Huang Lian Jie Du Tang*
> *Xie Xin Tang (H. Lian, H. Qin, + Da Huang)*
> *Pu Ji Xiao Du Yin*

Formulas:

Clear Heat

Bai Hu Tang	*Xie Xin Tang*	*Dao Chi San*
Zhu Ye Shi Gao Tang	*Pu Ji Xiao Du Yin*	**Long Dan Xie Gan Tang**
Qing Ying Tang	**Ma Xing Shi Gan Tang**	*Bai Tou Weng Tang*
Xi Jiao Di Huang Tang	*Xie Bai San*	**Qing Hao Bie Jia Tang**
Huang Lian Jie Du Tang	*Xie Huang San*	*Liu Yi San*

4 Levels Formulas (Wen Bing)
1. Lu/St **Qi Level** Heat w/ injured fluids:
2. Blazing Yang Ming *Channel* Heat/**Qi Level**:
(vs. what formula for Yang Ming *Organ* Heat:)
3. **Ying Level** Heat:
4. **Blood Level** Heat:

5. **Deficient Heat** (smoldering in the yin regions of the body):
6. **Summer Heat** (disturbing the Heart):

Heat Toxin
7. Acute, massive **febrile disorder of the head due to seasonal epidemic toxin** associated with W/H & Damp Phlegm:
8. Severe obstruction of the **three burners** by fire toxin, pervading both the interior and exterior:

Clear Organ Heat
9. Smoldering Fire due to constrained Heat in the **Lungs**:
(emphasis is on Draining Heat to stop wheezing)

10. Heat lodged in the **Lungs** obstructing the flow of qi:
(emphasis is on Regulating Lung Qi to stop wheezing)

11. Heat in the **Heart and Small Intestine channels**:
12. Smoldering Fire in the **Spleen**:
13. Heat Excess in the **Liver and/or Gallbladder channels**:
14. Heat Toxin searing the **Stomach and Intestines**:

Bai Hu Tang	*Huang Lian Jie Du Tang*	*Ma Xing Shi Gan Tang*	*Qing Hao Bie Jia Tang*
1.	1.	1.	1.
2.	2.	2.	2.
3.	3.	3.	3.
4.	4.	4.	4.
		Dx: ext w/c or w/h transf. to Lung Heat	5.

Long Dan Xie Gan Tang

Excess Liv/GB Heat (title herb):	Promote urination:	Protect the Yin/Clear Heat:
1.	4.	8.
Clear D/H	5.	Protect the Blood:
2.	6.	9.
3.	Move Liv Qi & Tx Shao Yang:	Harmonize the Middle:
	7.	10.

1. **Night fever** and morning coolness with an absence of sweating as the fever recedes, **emaciation** with no loss of appetite, **red tongue with little coating, and a fine, rapid pulse.**
Formula:

2. **Irritability with a sensation of heat in the chest**, thirst with a desire to drink cold beverages, a red face, possibly **sores around the mouth**, a red tongue, and a rapid pulse. (possibly also **dark, scanty, rough, and painful urination**, or visible blood in urine).
Formula:

3. **Pain in the hypochondria, headache, dizziness, red and sore eyes,** hearing loss, swelling in the ears, a bitter taste in the mouth, irritability, **short temper, a wiry rapid and forceful pulse and a red tongue with a yellow coating.**
Formula:

4. **Difficult and painful urination** with a sensation of heat in the urethra, **swollen and pruritic external genitalia, or foul smelling leukorrhea.** Shortened menstrual cycle with reddish-purple blood. A wiry rapid and forceful pulse and a red tongue with a yellow coating.
Formula:

5. Mouth ulcers, bad breath, thirst, frequent hunger, dry mouth and lips, a red tongue and a rapid pulse. (Also for tongue thrusting in children).
Formula:

6. **Strong fever and chills, redness, swelling and burning pain of the head and face,** dysfunction of the throat, dryness and **thirst**, and red tongue with a powdery-white or yellow coating, and a floating rapid and forceful pulse. (sudden onset)
Formula:

7. **High fever, irritability**, a dry mouth and throat, **incoherent speech, insomnia,** dark urine, a red tongue with a yellow coating, and a rapid, forceful pulse. (Also for **nosebleed or vomiting of blood** due to heat excess carbuncles, deep-rooted boils, and other toxic swelling and dysenteric disorders or jaundice due to damp-heat)
Formula:

8. **Fever, various types of bleeding** (including vomiting blood, nosebleed, blood in the stool or urine, and rashes), black and tarry stools, abdominal distension and fullness, thirst with an inability to swallow, **a scarlet tongue with prickles,** and a **thin, rapid pulse. (possible delirium)**
Formula:

9. **High fever that worsens at night,** severe **irritability and restlessness**, a scarlet, dry tongue, and a thin, rapid pulse. (possible thirst, delirium, **faint indistinct erythema and purpura**).
Formula:

10. Lingering fever (from a febrile disease) accompanied by vomiting, irritability and thirst, **parched mouth, lips and throat**, a choking cough, stifling sensation in the chest, a red tongue with little coating, and a deficient, rapid pulse. (possible restlessness and insomnia).
Formula:

11. **High fever with profuse sweating** and an aversion to heat, a red face, **severe thirst** and irritability, and a **flooding, forceful or slippery rapid pulse.** May also include headache, toothache, or bleeding of the gums and nose.
Formula:

12. Fever, sweating, thirst, irritability, urinary difficulty, a thin, yellow and greasy tongue coating, and a soggy, rapid pulse.
Formula:

13. Fever, irritability and restlessness, flushed face, red eyes, dark urine, constipation, a greasy, yellow tongue coating, and in severe cases, delirious speech. Also for epigastric focal distension*, jaundice, diarrhea, and dysenteric disorder; or vomiting of blood or nosebleed; or red and swollen eyes and ears; or ulcerations of the tongue and mouth; or abscesses:
Formula:

*Focal Distension (*Pi Man*): Either subjective feeling of fullness and distress in the chest and abdomen due to obstruction of qi, or localized distension in the epigastrium (*xie xin*), often resembling an overturned cup, and accompanied by muscular weakness and atrophy.

Clumping (*jie*): 1. process of congealing in the body, occurring from heat, cold, or stagnation. If more than one pathogen is involved referred to as a 'complex' (i.e. heat-cold complex as in *Ban Xia Xie Xin Tang*) (also the term for nodules, and the slow-irregular or knotted pulse)

14. Fever with or without sweating, thirst, **wheezing,** coughing, **labored breathing, nasal flaring** and pain, a yellow tongue coating, and a slippery, rapid pulse.
Formula:

15. Coughing, wheezing, and fever with skin that feels hot to the touch, all of which worsen in the late afternoon. Also dry mouth, little or difficult to expectorate sputum, a thin, rapid pulse, and a red tongue with a yellow coating.
Formula:

	Liu Wei Di Huang Tang	Qing Hao Bie Jia Tang
Jun Herb:	Shu Di Huang	Qing Hao, Bie Jia
Other Herbs:	Shan Zhu Yu, Shan Yao, Mu Dan Pi, Fu Ling, Ze Xie	Sheng Di, Zhi Mu, Mu Dan Pi
Sx:	hot flashes, night sweats	low-grade night fever
Emphasis:	Nourish Yin	Clear Deficient Heat

Heart- Hand Shao Yin

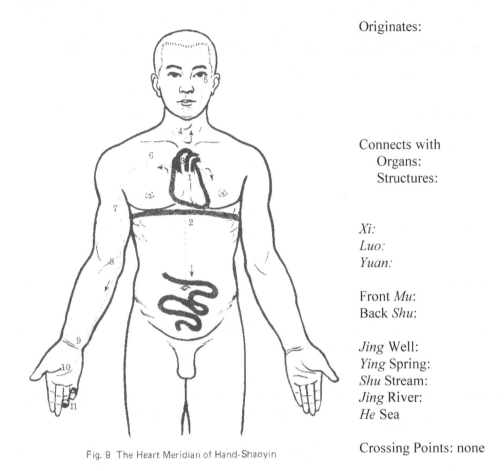

Fig. 9 The Heart Meridian of Hand-Shaoyin

Originates:

Connects with
    Organs:
    Structures:

Xi:
Luo:
Yuan:

Front *Mu:*
Back *Shu:*

Jing Well:
Ying Spring:
Shu Stream:
Jing River:
He Sea

Crossing Points: none

Channel Pathway
    This channel **begins in its associated organ, the Heart**, then emerges through the **blood vessel system surrounding the Heart**, and travels downward across the **diaphragm** where it connects with the **Small Intestine**.
    A **branch** of the main channel separates in the Heart and ascends alongside the **esophagus** to the face where it joins the **tissues surrounding the eye**.
    Another **branch** goes directly from the Heart to the **Lung**, then slants downward to emerge below the axilla. From here, the channel descends along the medial border of the anterior aspect of the upper arm, behind the Lung and Pericardium channels, to the antecubital fossa, where it continues downward to the capitate bone proximal to the palm. It then enters the palm and follows the medial side of the little finger to the finger tip.

Heart Channel Sx: general feverishness, headache, pain in the eyes, pain along the back of the upper arm, dry throat, thirst, hot or painful palms, coldness in the palms and soles of the feet, pain along the scapula and/or medial aspect of the forearm.

Heart Organ Sx: pain or fullness in chest and ribs or below ribs, irritability, shortness of breath, discomfort when reclining, vertigo, mental disorders

*Image from CAM, description from ACT

Small Intestine- Hand Tai Yang

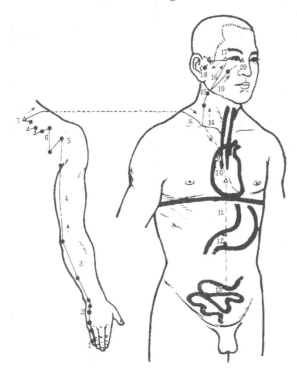

Fig. 10 The Small Intestine Meridian of Hand-Taiyang

Originates:

Connects with
  Organs:
  Structures:

Xi:
Luo:
Yuan:

Front *Mu:*
Back *Shu:*

Jing Well:
Ying Spring:
Shu Stream:
Jing River:
He Sea
Lower *He* Sea:

Confluent Point (8 extras):
  of channel:

Crossing Pts:

SI 12 crosses with:

Channel Pathway

This channel originates at the ulnar side of the tip of the little finger and ascends along the ulnar side of the hand to the wrist, emerging at the styloid process of the ulna. From here, it travels directly upward along the posterior aspect of the ulna, passing between the olecranon of the ulna and the medial epicondyle of the humerus at the medial side of the elbow. It then proceeds along the posterior border of the lateral aspect of the upper arm, emerging behind the shoulder joint and circling around the superior and inferior fossa of the scapula. At the top of the shoulder, it crosses the Bladder channel at points **UB 41** (*Fu Fen*) and **UB 11** (*Da Zhu*), and the Du channel at **Du 14** (*Da Zhui*), where the channel turns downward into the **supraclavicular fossa**, and connects with the **Heart**. From here, it descends along the **esophagus** and crosses the **diaphragm** to the **Stomach**. Before reaching its associated organ, the **Small Intestine**, the channel intersects the Ren (Conception) channel internally, and very deep, at points **Ren 13** (*Shang Wan*) and **Ren 12** (*Zhong Wan*).

A **branch** of this channel travels upward from the supraclavicular fossa and crosses the neck and cheek to the **outer canthus** of the eye, where it meets the Gall Bladder channel at **GB 1** (*Tong Zi Liao*). Then it turns back across the temple and enters the ear at point SI 19 (*Ting Gong*).

Another **branch** separates from the former branch on the cheek, ascends to the infraorbital region of the eye and then to the **inner canthus**, where it meets the Bladder channel at **UB 1** (*Jing Ming*). It then crosses horizontally to the zygomatic region.

According to chapter 4 of the *Ling Shu*, another **branch** descends to St 39 (*Xia Ju Xu*), the Lower Uniting Point (Lower *He Sea*) of the Small Intestine.

Small Intestine Channel Sx: numbness of the mouth and tongue, pain in the neck or cheek, sore throat, stiff neck, pain along the lateral aspect of the shoulder and upper arm.

Small Intestine Organ Sx: pain and distension in the lower abdomen, possibly extending around the waist or to the genitals; diarrhea, or abdominal pain with 'dry' stool or constipation.

*Image from CAM, description from ACT

HEART SYNDROMES

	Tongue	Pulse	Palpitations	Breathing	Sweating	Insomnia	Sleep	Dream Disturbed Sleep	Poor Memory	Other Sx
Heart Qi Def										
Heart Yang Def										
Heart Yang Exhaustion										
Heart Blood Def										
Heart Yin Def										
Heart Blood Stasis										
Phlegm Misting the Heart										
Heart Phlegm-Fire										

SMALL INTESTINE SYNDROMES

	Tongue	Pulse	Sx
Small Intestine Qi Disturbance			

Shu **Stream**
Indications:

Lu___   St___   Ht___   UB___   P ___   GB___
LI___   Sp___   SI___   K ___   SJ___   Liv___

1. Cough, asthma, hemoptysis, sore throat, palpitation, pain in the chest, wrist and arm:

2. Headache, redness of the eyes, **deafness, tinnitus,** sore throat, febrile diseases, pain in the elbow and arm, motor impairment of fingers:

3. Facial or general edema, abdominal pain, borborygumus, swelling and pain of the dorsum of the foot:

4. Sore throat, toothache, deafness, tinnitus, dizziness, spitting of blood, asthma, thirst, irregular menstruation, insomnia, nocturnal emission, impotence, frequency of micturition, pain in the lower back:

5. Toothache, opthalmalgia, sore throat, redness and swelling of fingers and the dorsum of the hand:

6. **Pain and rigidity of the neck**, tinnitus, deafness, sore throat, mania, malaria, **acute lumbar sprain, night sweating,** febrile diseases, contracture and numbness of the fingers, pain in the shoulder and elbow:

7. Gastric pain, abdominal distension, constipation, dysentery, vomiting, diarrhea, borborygmus, sluggishness, beriberi:

8. **Headache,** vertigo, pain of the outer canthus, scrofula, **pain in the hypochondriac region,** distending pain of the breast, **irregular menstruation**, pain and swelling of the dorsum of foot, spastic pain of the foot and toe:

9. Mania, headache, neck rigidity, blurring of vision, backache, pain in the lower extremities:

10. Headache, dizziness and vertigo, insomnia, congestion, swelling and pain of the eye, depression, **infantile convulsion, deviation of the mouth, pain in the hypochondriac region**, uterine bleeding, **hernia**, enuresis, retention of urine, epilepsy, pain in the anterior aspect of the medial malleolus:

11. **Cardiac pain, palpitation, stomachache, vomiting**, mental disorders, epilepsy, stuffy chest, pain in the hypochondriac region, convulsion, insomnia, irritability, foul breath:

12. Cardiac pain, irritability, palpitation, hysteria, amnesia, **insomnia**, mania, epilepsy, dementia, pain in the hypochondriac region, feverish sensation in the palm, yellowish sclera:

Jing **River**
Indications:

Lu___	St___	Ht___	UB___	P____	GB____
LI__	Sp__	SI__	K____	SJ____	Liv____

1. Migraine, pain of the outer canthus, pain in the axillary region, scrofula, lumbar pain, pain in the chest, hypochondriac region and lateral aspect of the lower extremities, malaria:

2. Cough, asthma, fever, pain the chest, sore throat, pain in the wrist:

3. Hernia, pain in the external genitalia, nocturnal emission, retention of urine, distending pain in the hypochondrium:

4. Abdominal distension, constipation, diarrhea, borborygmus, pain and rigidity of the tongue, pain in the foot and ankle, hemorrhoid:

5. **Cardiac pain, palpitation, stomachache, vomiting**, febrile diseases, irritability, malaria, mental disorders, epilepsy, swelling of the axilla, **contracture of the elbow and arm**:

6. Cardiac pain, spasmodic pain of elbow and arm, sudden loss of voice:

7. Headache, blurring of vision, neck rigidity, epistaxis, pain in the shoulder, back and arm, swelling and pain of the heel, **difficult labour**, epilepsy:

8. Headache, redness, pain and swelling of the eye, toothache, sore throat, pain of the wrist:

9. Edema, abdominal distension, diarrhea, borborygmus, muscular atrophy of the leg, **night sweating, spontaneous sweating, febrile diseases without sweating**:

10. Pain of the ankle joint, muscular atrophy, motor impairment, pain and paralysis of the lower extremities, epilepsy, headache, dizziness and vertigo, abdominal distension, constipation:

11. Swelling of the neck and sub-mandibular region, pain of the hand and wrist, febrile diseases:

12. Tinnitus, deafness, **pain in the hypchondriac region**, vomiting, **constipation**, febrile diseases, aching and heavy sensation of the shoulder and back, sudden hoarseness of voice:

QI 氣
1. essential substances of the human body (finest material substance)
2. functional activities of the zang-fu organs and tissues

6 Functions of Qi (CAM)
1.   4.
2.   5.
3.   6. Qi Hua

Yuan Qi (Source Qi)
Derived from/closely related to:
Supplemented by:
Root/origin:
Spreads to the body via:

Yuan Qi can be treated
1. needling *yuan*-source points
2. needling & moxa Ren points below the navel
3. needling & moxa *Ming Men*, Du 4

Gu Qi (Food Qi)
Food is "rotted & ripened" by the _____ and transformed into *Gu Qi* by the _____
Gu Qi combines with air in the Lung to produce:
Gu Qi goes to the Lungs, then to the Heart, and is transformed into:
      This process is facilitated by (type of Qi):

Zong Qi (Gathering Qi, Chest Qi, Ancestral Qi)
Combination of:
Functions:

Zhen Qi (True Qi)
Final transformation of Qi (facilitated by *Yuan Qi*)
Two forms:
1.
2.

Ying Qi 營氣 *(Nutritive Qi)*
Derived from:
Circulates (where):
Function:

Wei Qi 衛氣 *(Defensive Qi)*
Derived from:
Circulates (where):
Primary function:
Additional functions:
1.   3.
2.   4.

Additionally there is the qi of each Zang & Fu organ and meridian.

Zheng Qi 正氣 *(Upright Qi)*
General term to indicate the various kinds of Qi, usually used only in relation and contrast to Pathogenic Factor (*Xie Qi* 邪氣)

Zhong Qi 中氣 belongs to which organs:

BLOOD (*XUE* 血)
Derived from:
Function:
Material foundation for/houses and anchors:
What kind of Qi circulates with Blood:

4 Aspects of Blood-Qi Relationship
    1.
    2.
    3.
    4.

ESSENCE (*JING* 精)
Stored:
Controls:
Men's Essence flows in_____ year cycles
Women's Essence flows in _____ year cycles

BODY FLUIDS (*JIN YE* 津液)
Originate from (what substance):
Clean part goes:

Dirty Part goes:

3 Zang organs involved with Body Fluids/Water Metabolism:
Source of Body Fluids (Fu Organ):

Thin, watery, circulate with *Wei Qi*:
Function:

Turbid, heavy, dense, circulate with *Ying Qi*:
Function:

Qi Pathology
1.   3.
2.   4.

Blood Pathology
    1.
    2.
    3.

CLEAR DAMP HEAT

herb (yao 藥)	flavor (wei 味)	temp (qi 氣)	channels								
huang qin	**bitter**	**cold**	**GB**	**LI**	Lu	**St**					
huang lian	**bitter**	**cold**		**LI**		St	Ht	**Liv**			
huang bai	**bitter**	**cold**							K	UB	
long dan cao	**bitter**	**cold**	**GB**			St		**Liv**			
ku shen	**bitter**	**cold**		**LI**			Ht	**Liv**		UB	SI
qin pi	**bitter**	**cold**	**GB**	**LI**		St		**Liv**			
hu huang lian	**bitter**	**cold**	**GB**	**LI**		St		**Liv**			

DRAIN DOWNWARD

herb (yao 藥)	flavor (wei 味)		temp (qi 氣)	channels							
PURGATIVES:											
da huang	**bitter**		**cold**	Ht	**LI**	Liv	St				
mang xiao	**bitter**, acrid		**very cold**		**LI**		St				
fan xie ye	**bitter,** sweet		**cold**		**LI**						
lu hui	**bitter**		**cold**		**LI**	Liv	St				
MOIST LAXATIVES:											
huo ma ren	sweet		neutral		**LI**		St	Sp			
yu li ren	sweet, acrid, bitter		neutral		**LI**			Sp	SI		
HARSH EXPELLANTS:											
qian niu zi	acrid	**sl. toxic**	cold		**LI**				SI	K	Lu
gan sui	bitter, sweet	**toxic**	cold		**LI**					K	Lu
da ji	bitter, acrid	**toxic**	cold		**LI**					K	Lu
yuan hua	bitter, acrid	**toxic**	warm		**LI**					K	Lu
ba dou	acrid	**toxic**	hot		**LI**		St				Lu

EXPEL WIND DAMP

herb (yao 藥)	flavor (wei 味)		temp (qi 氣)	channels						
du huo	**bitter, acrid**		**warm**	**K**	UB					
qin jiao	**bitter, acrid**		sl. cold			GB	**Liv**	St		
wei ling xian	**acrid,** salty		**warm**		UB					
hai tong pi	**bitter, acrid**		neutral	**K**			**Liv**		Sp	
mu gua	sour		**sl. warm**				**Liv**		Sp	
can sha	sweet, **acrid**		**warm**				**Liv**	St	Sp	
sang zhi	**bitter,** sweet		sl. cold				**Liv**			
wu jia pi	**acrid, bitter,**		**warm**	**K**			**Liv**			
cang er zi	sweet, **sl. bitter**	toxic	**warm**							Lu
xi xian cao	**bitter**		cold	**K**			**Liv**			
bai hua she	sweet, salty	toxic	**warm**				**Liv**		Sp	
wu shao she	sweet, salty		neutral				**Liv**		Sp	
song jie	**bitter**		**warm**				**Liv**			

Herbs

Clear Damp Heat

Huang Qin   *Long Dan Cao*   Hu Huang Lian
Huang Lian   *Ku Shen*   *Bai Xian Pi* (also in Clear Toxic Heat)
Huang Bai   *Qin Pi*

1. _____ clears **yin deficient heat** and treats childhood nutritional impairment.

All three clear heat, dry dampness, drain fire and relieve toxicity. Commonly combined for mutual reinforcement.

2. _____ primarily **clears heat from the Lung**, also **calms the fetus**.

3. _____ mainly **drains fire from the Heart and Stomach**, also clears Damp Heat from the Stomach and Intestines.

4. _____ enters the Kidney to drain Deficient Fire, clears **Damp Heat from the   lower jiao.**

Both are for Liver Fire.

5. _____ benefits the eyes, treats Wind Damp Heat Bi, and bloody dysentery.

6. _____ is also for Liver Wind Heat & Damp Heat in the Liver & GB channels.

7. _____ **disperses wind, kills parasites**, and **stops itching**. Like *Huang Bai* and *Long Dan Cao*, this herb is used for damp heat in the lower jiao. Like *Huang Lian*, it clears heat and alleviates dysentery.

8. _____ is for **Wind Heat or Damp Heat** sores, carbuncles and rashes, marked by much pus, moist skin and pruritis. Additionally, it relieves toxicity, and in combination is used for Damp Heat jaundice or Bi syndrome.

Drain Downward

Purgatives	Moist Laxatives	Harsh Expellants (fluid)
Da Huang	*Huo Ma Ren*	*Qian Niu Zi*
Mang Xiao	*Yu Li Ren*	*Gan Sui*
Fan Xie Ye		*(Jing) Da Ji*
Lu Hui		*Yuan Hua*
		Ba Dou
		Shang Lu

Purgatives

1. _____ enters the Large Intestine channel only, drains downward and guides out stagnation for **constipation due to Heat** accumulating in the Intestines. Additionally, it **can be steeped as a tea** using only 1.5-3 grams (0.5-1 qian).

2. _____ has many functions, in part dependent on its preparation:
   Drains Heat and purges accumulation (fresh is strongest, add last 10 minutes of cooking)
   Drains Damp Heat via the stool and clears Heat in the Blood level.
   Drains Heat from the Blood causing bleeding (charred)
   Invigorates Blood, dispels stasis (wine or vinegar treated)
   Clears Heat, reduces Fire toxicity (topically or internally)

3. _____ clears heat and reduces swelling, purges accumulation and guides out stagnation. Dissolve into the strained decoction.

4. Besides draining fire and guiding out accumulation, _____, a relatively mild herb, also kills parasites, strengthens the Stomach, and cools the Liver.

Moist Laxatives

5. _____ moistens the Intestine/unblocks the bowel for **constipation due to Qi stagnation, and promotes urination and reduces edema**.
6. _____ moistens the Intestine for **constipation in the elderly, and with Blood deficiency**, it also **mildly nourishes the Yin**, and promotes the healing of sores (orally or topically)

Harsh Expellants (Cathartics for Fluid Stagnation)- (Some teachers do not cover this section)

7. _____ & _____ treat **Intestinal parasites**.

8. _____ & _____ **reduce swelling**.

9. _____ warms, unblocks and vigorously purges to treat edema, it bursts clogged phlegm and improves the condition of the throat, and treats abscesses and ulcers.

10. _____ drives out water through the urethra and anus (for edema with constipation) and reduces sores and carbuncles (fresh herb used topically).

Expel Wind Damp

Du Huo
Qin Jiao
Wei Ling Xian
Hai Tong Pi
Mu Gua
Can Sha
Sang Zhi
Hai Feng Teng
Cang Er Zi

Wu Jia Pi
(Cang Er Zi)
Xi Xian Cao
Luo Shi Teng
Hai Feng Teng
Qian Nian Jian
Hu Gu
Qian Nian Jian

Bai Hua She
Wu Shao She
She Tui
Song Jie
Fang Ji (Drain Damp)
Sang Ji Sheng (Tonify Yin)
Luo Shi Teng
Kuan Jin Teng

1. _____ effectively **dispels Wind Cold Damp in the lower half of the body**, also used for Shao Yin headache radiating to the teeth and cheeks. Can be used for acute or chronic, though generally used more for chronic conditions.

2. _____ dispels Wind, drains Damp Heat and unblocks the channels for **Wind Damp Heat Bi**. Additionally, it is sometimes put in the "Drain Damp" category because of its function of **promoting urination to reduce edema**.

3. _____ is bitter & neutral, and enters the Kidney & Liver channels. It **tonifies the Liver and Kidneys, strengthens the sinews and bones, and expels Wind Damp**. Additionally it nourishes Blood, **calms the fetus**, and benefits the skin.

4. _____ is bitter & cold, and also enters the Kidney & Liver channels. It can be used raw to treat **Damp Heat Bi** (and eczema , sores and ulcers), and steamed with wine to **tonify the Liver and Kidney**. Additionally it **calms the *shen* and pacifies the Liver.**

5. Commonly soaked in wine, _____ is primarily used to treat **Wind Damp Bi accompanied by weakness of the sinews and bones**. Additionally it promotes urination and reduces swelling.

6. Sweet, salty, warm and toxic, _____ **powerfully unblocks the channels and extinguishes Wind**. Also used to dispel Wind from the skin (rash or numbness) and sinews (tremors, seizures, paralysis). _____ has the same functions, although not as strong.

DUI YAO
Synergistic Herb Combinations

Da Huang & Mang Xiao
One frees the flow of stools.
The other softens the stools.
Combined they **purge Excess Heat
and Internal Accumulation
and purge the bowel.**
> *Da Cheng Qi Tang*
> *Tiao Wei Cheng Qi Tang*
> *Liang Ge San*
> *Tao He Cheng Qi tang*
> *Xin Jia Huang Long Tang*

Zhi Shi & Hou Po
Zhi Shi dissipates clumps and reduces focal distension.
Hou Po disseminates Qi and relieves the sensation of fullness.
Together they **promote bowel movement by moving Qi.**
> *Da Cheng Qi Tang*
> *Xiao Cheng Qi Tang*
> Ma Zi Ren Wan
> Zhi Shi Gua Lou Gui Zhi Tang

Da Cheng Qi Tang Ingredient Comparison:

Da Huang	Mang Xiao	Zhi Shi	Hou Po
Purges & Clears Heat	Softens Hardness	Breaks up & Descends Qi	Dries Damp, Moves Qi
Shi Hardness	*Zao* Dryness	*Pi* Distension (subjective)	*Man* Visible Bloating (objective)

Da Cheng Qi Tang
1. _da huang_
2. _mang xiao_
3. _zhi shi_
4. _hou po_
yang ming organ disorder

Xiao Cheng Qi Tang → **_Ma Zi Ren Wan_**
1. _da huang_   _Xiao Cheng Qi Tang_
2. _hou po_   _+ huo ma ren, xing ren, bai shao_
3. _zhi shi_   **_moistens intestine, drains heat_**
mild yang ming   **_moves qi, unblocks bowel_**
organ disorder

Tiao Wei Cheng Qi Tang → **_Tao He Cheng Qi Tang_** → **_Liang Ge San_**
1. _da huang_   _Tiao Wei Cheng Qi Tang_   _Tiao Wei Cheng Qi T._
2. _mang xiao_   _+ tao ren, gui zhi_   _+ huang qin, zhi zi, lian qiao_
3. _gan cao_   **_drains heat &_**   _bo he, zhu ye_
mild constipation due to   **_breaks up blood stasis_**   **_heat, irritability in_**
yang ming organ heat   **_chest & abdomen_**

Zeng Ye Tang → **_Zeng Ye Cheng Qi Tang_** → **_Xin Jia Huang Long Tang_**
1. _xuan shen_   _Zeng Ye Tang_   _Zeng Ye Tang_
2. _mai dong_   _+ da huang, mang xiao_   _+ Tiao Wei Cheng Qi Tang_
3. _sheng di_   **_yang ming organ disorder_**   _+ ren shen, dang gui, hai shen_
generates fluids,   **_with yin deficiency_**   **_enriches yin, augments qi_**
moistens dryness,   **_drains heat & purges_**
unblocks the bowel

Shi Zao Tang → **_Zhou Che Wan_**
1. _gan sui_   _Shi Zao Tang_
2. _jing da ji_   _+ qian niu zi, da huang, qing pi,_
3. _yuan hua_   _chen pi, bing lang, mu xiang, qing fen_
+ 10 _da zao_   **_moves qi, harshly drives out water_**
purges congested fluids   **_& heat accumulation_**

Formulas

Drain Downward

Da Cheng Qi Tang   *Da Xian Xiong Tang*   *San Wu Bei Ji Wan*
Xiao Cheng Qi Tang   *Xin Jia Huang Long Tang* *Shi Zao Tang*
Tiao Wei Cheng Qi Tang *Ma Zi Ren Wan*   *Zhou Che Wan*
Zeng Ye Cheng Qi Tang *Ji Chuan Jian*
Liang Ge San   Da Huang Fu Zi Tang

Purge Heat Accumulation
1. Vigorously purges heat accumulation (which is taking form)
Focal distension, fullness, dryness and hardness:

2. Moderately purges clumped heat
Focal distension, fullness, hardness (no dryness):

3. Mildly purges clumped heat,
for mild constipation due to Yang Ming stage heat:
Focal distension or fullness:

4. Enrich in generate fluids, drain heat & unblock the bowel:

5. Unformed Heat above, and formed accumulation below:

6. Heat and internal accumulation of water and fluids clumping in the chest:

7. Enrich Yin augment qi, drain heat and purge:

Moisten the Intestine, Unblock the Bowel
8. Moisten the intestines, drain heat, move qi, unblock the bowels:

9. Warm the Kidneys, moisten the intestines, unblock the bowel:

Warm the Yang, Guide Out Accumulation
10. Warm the interior, disperse cold, unblock the bowels, alleviate pain:

11. Harshly purge cold accumulation:

Drive Out Excess Water
12. Congested fluids in the chest and hypochondriac regions (cough with chest pain & hard focal distension):

13. Moves qi & harshly drives out water and heat accumulation:

Da Cheng Qi Tang	Xiao Cheng Qi Tang	Tiao Wei Cheng Qi Tang
1.	1.	1.
2.	2.	2.
3.	3.	3.
4.		

Urinary Bladder- Foot Tai Yang

Originates:

Connects with
  Organs:
  Structures:

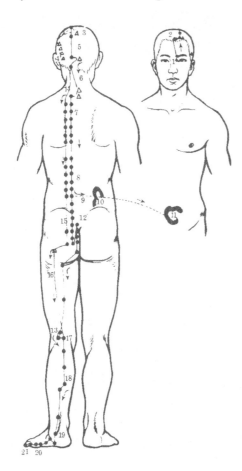

Xi:

Luo:

Yuan:

Front *Mu*:
Back *Shu*:

Jing Well:
Ying Spring:
Shu Stream:
Jing River:
He Sea

Lower *He* Sea of SJ:

Confluent Point (8 extras):
  of which channel:

Yang Qiao *Xi* Cleft:

Promote Labor Pts:
(contraindicated in pregnancy)

Influential point of Bones:
Influential point of Blood:
Command point (& area):

Crossing Points:

Fig. 11 The Bladder Meridian of Foot-Taiyang

Channel Pathway

This channel begins at **UB 1** (*Jing Ming*) at the **inner canthus** of the eye and ascends across the forehead, intersecting the Governing channel at **Du 24** (*Shen Ting*), and the Gall bladder channel at point **GB 15** (*Tou Lin Qi*). It then crosses to the **vertex** and again intersects the Governing channel at point **Du 20** (*Bai Hui*).

From here, a **branch** descends to the area above the ear, joining the Gall Bladder channel at points **GB 7** (*Qu Bin*), **GB 8** (*Shuai Gu*)**, GB 12** (*Wan Gu*), etc.

A vertical **branch** enters the **brain** at the vertex and intersects with the Governing channel at **Du 17** (*Nao Hu*), before emerging and descending along the nape of the neck and the muscles of the medial scapula. Here the Bladder channel meets the Governing channel at points **Du 14** (*Da Zhui*) and **Du 13** (*Tao Dao*), after which it continues downward, parallel to the spine, to the lumbar region. The channel then enters the internal cavity via the paravertebral muscles, communicates with the **Kidneys**, and finally joins its associated Organ, the **Bladder.**

Yet another **branch** separates from the main channel at the back of the neck and descends, parallel to the spine, from the medial side of the scapula to the gluteal region. Here it crosses the buttock to intersect the Gall Bladder channel at point **GB 30** (*Huan Tiao*), and then descends across the lateral posterior aspect of the thigh to join with the other branch of this channel in the popliteal fossa. Continuing downward through the gastrocnemius muscle, the channel emerges behind the external malleolus, then follows the 5th metatarsal bone, crossing its tuberosity to the lateral tip of the little toe at point **UB 67** (*Zhi Yin*).

According to chapter 4 of the *Ling Shu,* the Bladder channel connects behind the knee with its Lower Uniting point, **UB 40** (*Wei Zhong*).

U.B. Channel Sx: alternating chills and fever, headache, stiff neck, pain in the lumbar region, nasal congestion, disease of the eye, pain along the back of the leg and foot.

U.B. Organ Sx: pain in the lower abdomen, enuresis, retention of urine, painful urination, mental disorders.

*Image from CAM, description from ACT

Kidney- Foot Shao Yin

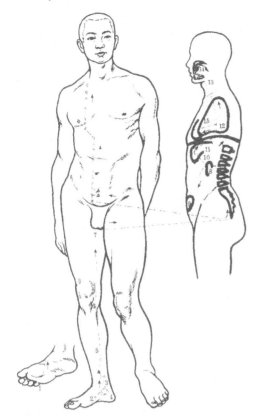

Fig. 12 The Kidney Meridian of Foot Shaoyin

Originates:

Connects with
  Organs:
  Structures:

Xi:
Luo:
Yuan:

(Front) *Mu*:
Back *Shu:*

Jing Well:
Ying Spring:
Shu Stream:
Jing River:
He Sea

Confluent Point (8 extras):
  of which channel:

Yin Qiao *Xi* Cleft:
Yin Wei Xi Cleft:

Crossing Pts:

Channel Pathway

This channel begins beneath the little toe, crosses the sole of the foot and emerges at point **K 2** (*Ran Gu*) on the inferior aspect of the navicular tuberosity at the instep. From here it travels posterior to the medial malleolus, enters the heel, and proceeds upward along the medial aspect of the lower leg where it intersects the Spleen channel at point **Sp 6** (*San Yin Jiao*). Continuing up the leg within the gastrocnemius muscle, the channel traverses the medial aspect of the popliteal fossa and the medial, posterior aspect of the thigh to the base of the spine, where it intersects the Governing channel at **Du 1**(*Chang Qiang*). Here, it threads its way beneath the spine to enter its associated Organ, the **Kidney**, and to communicate with the **Bladder**. It intersects the Conception channel at points **Ren 4** (*Guan Yuan*) and **Ren 3** (*Zhong Ji*).

A **branch** ascends directly from the Kidney, crosses the **Liver** and **diaphragm**, enters the **Lung**, and follows the throat to the **root of the tongue.**

Another **branch** separates in the Lung**,** connects with the **Heart,** and disperses in the chest.

Kidney Channel Sx: pain along the lower vertebrae, low back pain, coldness in the feet, motor impairment or muscular atrophy of the foot, dryness in the mouth, sore throat, pain in the sole of the foot or along the posterior aspect of the lower leg or thigh.

Kidney Organ Sx: vertigo, facial edema, ashen complexion, blurred vision, shortness of breath, drowsiness and irritability, loose stool, chronic diarrhea or constipation, abdominal distension, vomiting, impotence.

*Image from CAM, description from ACT

KIDNEY SYNDROMES

	Tongue	Pulse	Sore Low Back & Knees	Urination	Male Sx	Female Sx	Dizziness	SOB	Other Sx.
Kidney Qi Def									
Kidney Yang Def									
Kidney Yin Def									

URINARY BLADDER SYNDROMES

	Tongue	Pulse	Sx
Urinary Bladder Damp Heat			

He **Sea Points**
Indications:

Lu___   St___   Ht___   UB___   P____   GB____
LI___   Sp__   SI__   K____   SJ____   Liv____

1. Cough, hemoptysis, afternoon fever, asthma, sore throat, fullness in the chest, infantile convulsions, spasmodic pain of the elbow and arm, mastitis: (no moxa)

2. Cardiac pain, spasmodic pain and numbness of the hand and arm, tremor of the hand, scrofula, pain in the axilla and hypochondriac region:

3. Headache, swelling of the cheek, pain in the nape, shoulder, arm and elbow, epilepsy:
Needling this point be careful of: _____

4. **Gastric pain**, vomiting, hiccup, abdominal distension, borborygmus, diarrhea, dysentery, constipation, mastitis, enteritis, aching of the knee joint and leg, beriberi, edema, cough, **asthma, emaciation due to general deficiency**, indigestion, apoplexy, **hemiplegia**, dizziness, insomnia, mania:
(Apoplexy: sudden inability to feel and move caused by blockage or rupture of an artery in the brain)

5. Impotence, hernia, uterine bleeding, dysuria, pain in the knee and popliteal fossa, mental disorders:
(between the tendons of _____ and _____)

6. **Sore throat,** toothache, redness and pain of the eye, scrofula, **urticaria**, motor impairment of the upper extremities, abdominal pain, vomiting, diarrhea, **febrile diseases:**

7. **Cardiac pain, palpitation**, febrile diseases, irritability, **stomachache, vomiting**, pain in the elbow and arm, tremor of the hand and arm:

8. Migraine, pain in the neck, shoulder and arm, epilepsy, scrofula, goiter:

9. **Hemiplegia, weakness, numbness and pain of the lower extremities,** swelling and pain of the knee, beriberi, hypochondriac pain, bitter taste in the mouth, vomiting, jaundice, infantile convulsion:

10. Prolapse of uterus, lower abdominal pain, retention of urine, nocturnal emission, pain in the external genitalia, pruritus vulvae, pain in the medial aspect of the knee and thigh:

11. **Low back pain**, motor impairment of the hip joint, contracture of the tendons in the popliteal fossa, muscular atrophy, pain, numbness and motor impairment of the lower extremities, hemiplegia, abdominal pain, vomiting, diarrhea, **erysipelas*:**

*Erysipelas: inflammation of the skin caused by a of type bacterium.

12. Abdominal pain and distension, diarrhea, dysentery, **edema,** jaundice, **dysuria, enuresis, incontinence of urine,** pain in the external genitalia, dysmenorrhea, pain in the knee:

Luo *Points*

How many *Luo* points are there?_____

Lu___   St___   Ht___   UB___   P___   GB____
LI___   Sp___   SI___   K____   SJ____   Liv____

+ 3 more: _____   _____   _____

1. **Cardiac pain,** palpitation, stuffy chest, pain in the hypochondriac region, **stomachache, nausea,** vomiting, hiccup, mental disorders, epilepsy, insomnia, febrile diseases , irritability, malaria, contracture and pain of the elbow and arm:
(between the tendons of _____ and _____)

2. Pain in the knee, muscular atrophy, motor impairment and pain of the lower extremities, **blurring of vision, opthalmalgia, night blindness**, distending pain of the breast:

3. Retention of urine, enuresis, hernia, irregular menstruation, leukorrhea, pruritus vulvae, weakness and atrophy of the leg:

4. Headache, dizziness and vertigo, cough, asthma, **excessive sputum**, pain in the chest, constipation, mania, epilepsy, muscular atrophy, motor impairment, pain, swelling or paralysis of the lower extremities:

5. Headache, blurring of vision, nasal obstruction, epistaxis, back pain, hemorrhoids, **weakness of the leg**:

6. Redness of the eye, tinnitus, deafness, epistaxis, aching of the hand and arm, sore throat, edema:

7. Headache, migraine, neck rigidity, cough, asthma, sore throat, facial paralysis, **toothache,** pain and weakness of the wrist:

8. Neck rigidity, headache, dizziness, spasmodic pain in the elbow and fingers, febrile diseases, mania:

9. Palpitation, dizziness, blurring of vision, sore throat, **sudden loss of voice, aphasia with stiffness of the tongue,** pain in the wrist and elbow:

10. Gastric pain, vomiting, abdominal pain and distension, diarrhea, dysentery, borborygmus:

11. Spitting of blood, asthma, stiffness and pain of the lower back, dysuria, constipation, pain in the heel, dementia:

12. Febrile diseases, headache, pain in the cheek, strained neck, deafness, tinnitus, pain in the hypochondriac region, motor impairment of the elbow and arm, pain of the fingers, hand tremor:

13. Pain in the chest and hypochondriac region, asthma, **general aching and weakness:**

14. Diarrhea, bloody stools, hemorrhoids, prolapse of the rectum, constipation, pain in the lower back, epilepsy:

15. Pain in the cardiac region and the chest, nausea, mental disorders, epilepsy:

Eight Principles:
Comparing Cold & Heat, Excess & Deficiency

Syndrome:	Cold	Heat
thirst	no	yes
complexion	pale	red
temperature of extremities	cold	warm
bowel movement	loose/diarrhea	constipation (dysentery)
urine	clear, copious	yellow, scanty
tongue	pale, moist white coat	red, yellow coat
pulse	slow	rapid

Syndrome:	External Cold	Internal Cold
character	acute, short, mild	chronic, long, severe
symptoms	slight fever, headache,	no fever, cold limbs,
	body ache, no sweating	copious urine, loose stool
	not relieved by covering up	relieved by covering up
tongue body	normal	pale
tongue coat	thin white (normal)	moist white
	floating & tight	deep, slow or tight

Syndrome	Excess Cold	Yang Deficient Cold
character	acute, short, severe	chronic, weak constitution
abdominal pain	worse with pressure	relieved by pressure
diarrhea	yes	in the morning
tongue coat	thick white	thin white
pulse	slow tight	slow deep
other	profuse sputum	fatigue, low back pain,

	Excess Heat	(Yin) Deficient Heat
general characteristics:	abrupt onset, acute, severe	slow onset, chronic,
	and rapid changes	slow changes
fever	high fever	low grade tidal fever
complexion	whole face red	red cheeks
thirst	for cold water	for warm water
sweating	day time sweating	night time sweating
heat feelings	whole body	fiver center heat
tongue	red with yellow coat	red with scanty coat
pulse	rapid forceful	rapid thready/thin

Differentiating Exterior Syndromes: Key Symptoms

Exterior General Sx:
> tongue coat:
> pulse:

External Cold Sx (W/C):
> tongue coat:
> pulse:

External Heat (W/H):
> tongue coat:
> pulse:

External Deficient Cold: **vs.**   **External Excess Cold:**

(Fever with aversion to Cold=Exterior syndrome)

<u>Interior</u>
1. Transmission of External pathogen to Interior
2. External pathogen directly invades Interior
3. Zang Fu functional disturbance (emotions, diet, overstrain, stress)

Pulse: Deep

Change in tongue body color or shape
*For details of Interior syndromes, see deficiency and excess, and also syndromes according to Zang Fu Dx (charts from first six weeks).

Complicated Syndromes of Heat & Cold
(True Heat & False Cold / True Cold & False Heat / Heat Above & Cold Below)

1. Sx: above: suffocation and heat sensation in the chest, frequent desire to vomit
   below: abdominal pain which can be alleviated by warmth, loose stools
Dx:

2. Sx: Cold limbs, burning sensation in the chest and abdomen, no aversion to cold, aversion to heat, thirst with preference for cold drinks, irritability, dry throat, foul breath, scanty deep yellow urine, constipation
P: deep, forceful
T: deep red tongue with yellow dry coating
Dx:

3. Sx: feverishness, flushed face, thirst for warm drinks, patient wants to cover up, clear urine, loose stools
P: superficial, weak
T: pale with white coating
Dx:

AROMATICALLY TRANSFORM DAMP

herb (yao 藥)	flavor (wei 味)		temp (qi 氣)	Channels			
Huo Xiang	acrid		sl. warm	Lu	Sp	St	
Pei Lan	acrid		neutral		Sp	St	
Hou Po	bitter, acrid	aromatic	warm	Lu	Sp	St	LI
Cang Zhu	acrid, bitter	aromatic	warm		Sp	St	
Bai Dou Kou	acrid	aromatic	warm	Lu	Sp	St	
Cao Dou Kou	acrid	aromatic	warm		Sp	St	
Cao Guo	acrid		warm		Sp	St	
Sha Ren	acrid	aromatic	warm		Sp	St	

DRAIN DAMP

herb (yao 藥)	flavor (wei 味)	temp (qi 氣)	Channels								
Fu Ling	sweet, bland	neutral	Ht	Sp	Lu						
Zhu Ling	sweet, bland	sl. cool		Sp		K	UB				
Hua Shi	sweet, bland	cold					UB	St			
Yi Yi Ren	sweet, bland	sl. cold		Sp	Lu	K					
Dong Gua Ren	sweet	cold			Lu			St	SI	LI	
Mu Tong	bitter	cool	Ht				UB		SI		
Tong Cao	sweet, bland	sl. cold			Lu			St			
Deng Xin Cao	sweet, bland	sl. cold	Ht		Lu				SI		
Qu Mai	bitter	cold	Ht				UB		SI		
Di Fu Zi	sweet, bitter	cold					UB				
Bian Xu	bitter	sl. cold					UB				
Shi Wei	bitter, sweet	sl. cold			Lu		UB				
Che Qian Zi	sweet	cold			Lu	K	UB			Liv	
Che Qian Cao	sweet	cold									
Dong Kui Zi	sweet	cold					UB		SI	LI	
Bei Xie	bitter	neutral					UB	St		Liv	
Jin Qian Cao	sweet, bland	neutral				K	UB			Liv	GB
Chi Xiao Dou	sweet, sour	neutral	Ht						SI		
Ze Xie	sweet, bland	cold				K	UB				
Yin Chen Hao	bitter, acrid	cool		Sp				St		Liv	GB
Han Fang Ji	bitter, acrid	cold		Sp		K	UB				
Yu Mi Xu	sweet	neutral					UB			Liv	GB

WARM THE INTERIOR

herb (yao 藥)	flavor (wei 味)		temp (qi 氣)	Channels					
Fu Zi	acrid	toxic	hot	Ht	K	Sp			
Gan Jiang	acrid		hot	Ht		Sp	St	Lu	
Rou Gui	acrid, sweet		hot	Ht	K	Sp		Liv	
Wu Zhu Yu	acrid, bitter	sl. toxic	hot		K	Sp	St	Liv	
Chuan Jiao	acrid	sl. toxic	hot		K	Sp	St		
Ding Xiang	acrid		warm		K	Sp	St		
Xiao Hui Xiang	acrid		warm		K	Sp	St	Liv	
Gao Liang Jiang	acrid		hot			Sp	St		
Bi Ba	acrid		hot				St		LI
Hu Jiao	acrid		hot				St		LI

Herbs
Aromatically Transform Damp

Huo Xiang	*(Bai Dou Kou)*
Pei Lan	*Cao Dou Kou*
Hou Po	*Cao Guo*
Cang Zhu	*Sha Ren*

All four herbs (related to cardamom) share the basic functions of transforming Dampness and facilitating the flow of Qi. In order from left to right the strength of transforming Dampness increases while facilitating flow of Qi decreases. Therefore the herb on the far right has the strongest function of transforming Dampness, while the herb on the far left has the best effect in facilitating the movement of Qi.

1. _____ 2. _____ 3. _____ 4. _____
(strongest at moving Qi…………………………………… strongest at transforming Damp)
(mildest at transforming Damp…………………………..mildest at moving Qi)
from Dafang Zeng's little blue & white book "Essentials of Chinese Medicine: Materia Medica

5. **The primary herb for Dampness accumulating in the Middle Jiao** with epigastric and abdominal distension, _____ also releases the exterior for Wind Cold and treats Wind Cold Damp Bi. Additionally it enhances visual acuity.

6. **The primary herb for reducing distension and eliminating fullness,** _____ may be combined with:
Cang Zhu for Damp obstruction and Qi stagnation,
Ban Xia to treat Phlegm with constrained Qi, or
Zhi Shi for fecal impaction due to Heat accumulation.

7. _____ is **the primary herb for Summer Heat Dampness** with aversion to Cold, fever, focal distension, vomiting and diarrhea. It harmonizes the Middle Jiao and is acrid to release the Exterior.

8. Like *Huo Xiang,* _____ treats Summer Heat Damp as well as turbid Dampness that lingers in the Middle Jiao. Often combined with *Huo Xiang*.

Huo Xiang	**Zi Su Ye**
Both dispel pathogens & release the exterior, Facilitate the flow of Qi & Harmonize the Middle	
Stronger aromatic and drying properties to Dry Damp & Stop Vomiting	Stronger acrid & dispersing qualities to Induce Perspiration and Disperse Cold

Drain Damp

Fu Ling	Deng Xin Cao	Dong Kui Zi
Zhu Ling	Qu Mai	Bei Xie
Hua Shi	Di Fu Zi	Jin Qian Cao
Yi Yi Ren	Bian Xu	Chi Xiao Dou
Dong Gua Ren	Shi Wei	Ze Xie
Mu Tong	Che Qian Zi	Yin Chen Hao
Tong Cao	Che Qian Cao	(Han Fang Ji)

1. Sweet, bland and neutral, _____ exclusively promotes urination and reduces edema without having any tonifying effect, (unlike *Fu Ling* which strengthens the Spleen).

2. _____ , the **Imperial herb for Spleen deficiency with excessive Dampness** causing congested fluids, edema and diarrhea. It is sweet, bland, and neutral, mildly strengthens the Spleen and quiets the Heart to calm the *Shen*.

3. _____ eliminates Damp Heat via urination. It treats Painful *Lin* syndrome and diarrhea. It has a unique characteristic of unblocking the water passage and separating the clear from the turbid. It is used to **treat watery diarrhea due to Dampness, by "promoting urination to solidify the bowel movement"**

4. Contraindicated in pregnancy, and to be used with caution (as acute renal failure may result from overdose) _____ promotes urination, for Heart Fire and S.I./UB Dampness, and also promotes lactation.

5. Similar to the herb in question 4., _____ also promotes urination and lactation, but is only cautioned in pregnancy.

6. _____ promotes urination, **relieves Summer Heat**, and can be applied topically for skin Dampness, such as eczema.

7. _____ separates the clear from the turbid, and is used specifically for **turbid Dampness causing cloudy urination**. Also can be used for Wind Damp Bi syndrome.

8. Milder than *Mu Tong* and *Tong Cao* in its promoting urination function, _____ **additionally enters the Heart channel** to clear Heart Heat and eliminate irritability.

9. Bitter, slightly cold, and entering the Liver, GB, Spleen and Stomach channels, _____ is the **Imperial herb for jaundice**, is appropriate for Yang type or Yin type depending on its combination with other herbs.

Shi Wei, Bian Xu, and *Qu Mai* all promote urination and unblock urinary tract obstruction for Heat *Lin* or Blood *Lin*. They are often combined for mutual reinforcement.
10. _____ is used externally for parasites and itching.
11. _____ invigorates Blood and facilitates menstrual flow.
12. _____ clears Heat from the Lung and stops coughing.

13. Sweet, bland and cold, _____ **drains both Yin Deficient Heat and Damp Heat.**

14. _____ **relieves toxicity and promotes purulent discharge** (may be applied topically). It promotes urination to reduce swelling, and drains Dampness for Damp Heat jaundice. Additionally it is a food.

15. Besides mildly promoting urination and clearing Heat, _____ is more effective in **stopping itching** due to Dampness **(both internally and as a wash)**

16. The Imperial herb for both **GB and Kidney stones** (used with *Ji Nei Jin*), _____ can also be applied topically to relieve toxicity and reduce swelling.

Warm the Interior

Fu Zi	*Chuan Jiao (aka Hua Jiao)*	*Bi Ba*
Gan Jiang	*Ding Xiang*	*Hu Jiao*
Rou Gui	*Xiao Hui Xiang*	
Wu Zhu Yu	*Gao Liang Jiang*	

Often combined, the following two herbs both warm the interior and dispel cold, tonify the fire and assist Yang.
1. Gentler than but longer lasting effects, _____ is the **Imperial herb for leading fire back to its source.** It is acrid, sweet, and hot and enters the Heart, Spleen, Liver and Kidney.
2. Acrid, hot and toxic, _____ is the **Imperial herb to tonify the fire and disperse cold, as well as restore devastated Yang**. It enters the Heart, Kidney, and Spleen, but is said to act on all 12 channels.

3. Besides warming the middle to disperse Cold and alleviate pain, _____ also eradicates roundworms.

Both of the following two herbs enter the Spleen and Stomach to warm the middle and disperse Cold.
4. _____ is the **Imperial herb for cold lodged in the Liver channel** (Lower Jiao). It also redirects Stomach Qi downward, and although it is hot can be combined with *Huang Lian* to treat Liver fire invading the Stomach.
5. _____ enters the Lung (Upper Jiao) to **warm the Lung and transform congested fluids**.

The following two herbs disperse Cold, facilitate the movement of Qi, worm the middle and descend rebellious Qi to treat vomiting. (They are both Indian spices as well).
6. _____ mainly enters the Liver channel and is the **Imperial herb for Cold hernia** disorder.
7. _____ also enters the Kidney channel to **warm the Kidney and assist Yang for impotence**. It is antagonized by *Yu Jin*.

8. _____ warms the middle, disperses Cold from the Stomach and Large Intestine, and alleviates pain. Additionally it can be applied topically as a powder for toothache..

9. _____ , also a spice, warms the middle and disperse Cold.

10. Both already mentioned in questions above, _____ & _____ **enter the Liver channel to treat hernia**?

Caution during Pregnancy: Contraindicated during Pregnancy:
Rou Gui   *Fu Zi*
Chuan Jiao

DUI YAO
Synergistic Herb Combinations

Bai Shao & Chai Hu
One is sour and astringent.
The other is acrid and dissipating.
Together they drain the Liver without damaging Liver Yin,
And nourish the Liver without causing Liver Qi Stagnation.
They regulate the Spleen and stop pain,
Harmonize the exterior and interior,
And constrain yin while upbearing Yang.
> *Si Ni San*
> *Xiao Yao San*

Chai Hu & Huang Qin
One dispels, upbears clear Yang, and expels External pathogens
The other drains, downbears turbidity and expels Internal pathogens.
Together they harmonize the Shao Yang,
The Interior and the Exterior, and the Liver and Gallbladder.
> *Xiao Chai Hu Tang*

Ban Xia & Huang Qin
One is warm, acrid and frees the flow.
The other is cold, bitter and drains.
Together they harmonize Yin and Yang, clear Heat and drain Fire,
Harmonize the Stomach and stop vomiting.
> *Xiao Chai Hu Tang*
> *Ban Xia Xie Xin Tang*

Bai Zhu & Fu Ling
One supplements, and dries.
The other leaches out Dampness and disinhibits urination
Together they supplement the Spleen and dry Dampness,
Leach out Dampness and disinhibit urination.

Si Jun Zi Tang	*Wu Ling San*
Liu Jun Zi Tang	*Huo Xiang Zheng Qi San*
Ba Zhen Tang	*Zhen Wu Tang*
Gui Pi Tang	*Etc.*
Shen Ling Bai Zhu San	

Formulas

Harmonizing

Xiao Chai Hu Tang　　　　　　*Gan Cao Xie Xin Tang*
Si Ni San　　　　　　　　　　*Sheng Jiang Xie Xin Tang*
Xiao Yao San　　　　　　　　*Huang Lian Tang*
Ban Xia Xie Xin Tang　　　　*(Shao Yao Gan Cao Tang: Tonify Blood)*

Harmonize Shao Yang:
1. Shao Yang Stage disorders:
2. What *Dui Yao* combination in the above formula addresses Shao Yang disorders? _____ &
_____

Harmonize Liver & Spleen
3. Liver constraint with Blood Deficiency:
4. Internal Heat constraining Yang Qi:

Harmonize Stomach & Intestine
5. Cold-Heat complex in the Middle Jiao (Exc & Def):

6. Alternating fever and chills, dry throat, bitter or sour taste, dizziness, irritability, chest/hypochondriac fullness, heartburn, n/v, reduced appetite.
T: thin, white coat
P: Wiry
Formula:
Herbs:
　　1.　　　　　　　5.
　　2.　　　　　　　6.
　　3.　　　　　　　7.
　　4.

7. Epigastric focal distension (*pi*), fullness and tightness with very slight or no pain, dry heaves or vomiting, borborygmus with diarrhea, reduced appetite.
T: thin, yellow, greasy coat
P: wiry, rapid
Formula:
Herbs:
　　1.　　　　　　　5.
　　2.　　　　　　　6.
　　3.　　　　　　　7.
　　4.

Variations of <u>Ban Xia Xie Xin Tang</u>:
8. In contrast, less intense heat, perhaps some remnant of an exterior condition.
Heat in the chest and Cold in the Stomach characterized by stifling sensation in the chest, irritability, nausea, abdominal pain, T: white greasy coat, P: wiry
(-*Huang Qin,* + *Gui Zhi*)
Formula:

9. More severe Stomach Qi Deficiency, with undigested food in stool & irritability;
Increase the dose to 4-5 *qian* (12-15 g) of:

Formula:

10. For water and Heat complex or Stomach Def with food stagnation and suspended fluids, characterized by firm epigastric focal distension, dry heaves with a foul odor, loud borborygmus and diarrhea.
Add 4 *qian* (12 g):
Formula:

11 & 12. There is a two-herb difference between **Xiao Chai Hu Tang**, which treats Shao Yang disorders, and **Ban Xia Xie Xin Tang**, which treats Heat-Cold Complex in the Middle Jiao.

Xiao Chai Hu Tang:	*Ban Xia Xie Xin Tang*
_____	_____
_____	_____
Huang Qin	*Huang Qin*
Ban Xia	*Ban Xia*
Ren Shen	*Ren Shen*
Da Zao	*Da Zao*
Zhi Gan Cao	*Zhi Gan Cao*

Xiao Yao San	**Si Ni San**
Liver:	1.
1.	2.
2.	3.
Spleen:	4.
3.	Main symptom:
4.	
Blood/Yin:	T:
5.	P:
6.	(There are no strong Heat symptoms, so
Harmonize:	the formula focuses on regulating & harmonizing)
7.	
8.	

13. Which *Dui Yao* herb combination in both of the above two formulas disseminates Liver Qi without injuring Liver Yin? _____ & _____

Treat Dryness

Xing Su San   *Bai He Gu Jin Tang*
Sang Xing Tang   *Mai Men Dong Tang*
Qing Zao Jiu Fei Tang   *Zeng Ye Tang*
Sha Shen Mai Men Dong Tang

Gently Disperse & Moisten Dryness
1. Warm Dryness (relatively Exterior):
2. Warm Dryness attacking Lungs causing rebellious Qi:
3. Cool Dryness (Externally contracted):
4. Dryness injuring Lungs and Stomach:

Enrich Yin & Moisten Dryness
5. Dry Intestines due to injured Fluids:
6. Internal Lung Dryness due to Lung & Kidney Yin Deficiency:
7. Deficiency Heat of the Stomach scorching the Lungs:

Xing Su San	*Bai He Gu Jin Tang*
Two title herbs:	Title herb:
1.	1.
2.	*Zeng Ye Tang* (nourish Yin, clear Heat)
Assistant to chief herbs:	2.
3.	3.
+ *Er Chen Tang*	4.
4.	Tonify Yin & Blood:
5.	5.
6.	6.
7.	7.
+ *Dui Yao:* up & down	Moisten Lung, transform phlegm (expensive):
8.	8.
9.	Guide to the Lungs, move Lung Qi, stop cough
+ the other 'two amigos'	9.
10.	Harmonize:
11.	10.

Pericardium- Hand Jue Yin

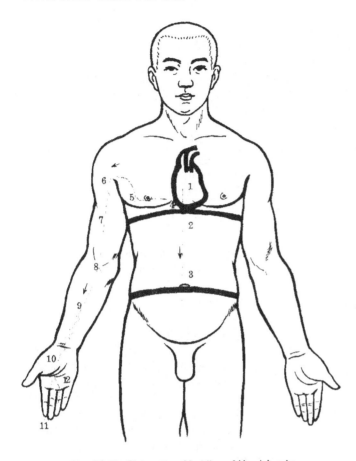

Originates:

Connects with
  Organs:
  Structures:

Xi:
Luo:
Yuan:

Front *Mu*:
Back *Shu*:

Jing Well:
Ying Spring:
Shu Stream:
Jing River:
He Sea

Confluent Point (8 extras):
  of which channel:

Crossing Points: none

Fig. 13 The Pericardium Meridian of Hand-Jueyin

Channel Pathway

This channel **begins in the chest** where it joins with its associated Organ, the **Pericardium**. It then descends across the **diaphragm** and into the abdomen, where it connects successively with the **upper, middle and lower burners of the Triple Burner.** ;

A **branch** of the main channel runs along the chest, emerging superficially in the costal region at point **P 1** (*Tian Chi*) three units below the anterior axillary fold before ascending to the inferior aspect of the axilla. From here, it descends along the medial aspect of the upper arm between the paths of the Lung and Heart channels to the antecubital fossa, and then proceeds down the forearm between the tendons of the **palmaris longus** and **flexor carpi radialis** muscles. Entering the palm, it follows the ulnar aspect of the middle finger until it reaches the finger tip.

Another **branch** separates in the palm and proceeds along the lateral aspect of the 4th finger to the finger tip (**SJ 1**).

Pericardium Channel Sx: stiff neck, spasms in the arm or leg, flushed face, pain in the eyes, subaxillary swelling, spasms and contracture of the elbow and arm, restricting movement, hot palms.

Pericardium Organ Sx: impaired speech, fainting, irritability, fullness in the chest, motor impairment of the tongue, palpitations, chest pain, mental disorders.

*Image from CAM, description from ACT

San Jiao- Hand Shao Yang

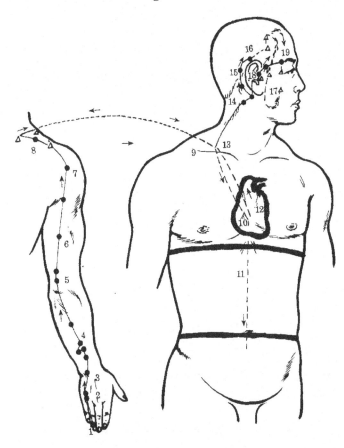

Fig. 14   The Triple Energizer Meridian of Hand-Shaoyang

Originates:

Connects with
   Organs:
   Structures:

Xi: Front *Mu:*
Luo: Back *Shu:*
Yuan:

Jing Well:
Ying Spring:
Shu Stream:
Jing River:
He Sea
Lower *He* Sea:

Confluent Pt (8 extras):
   of which channel:

Crossing Pts:

Channel Pathway

This channel originates on the ulnar aspect of the 4th finger tip, ascends between the 4th and 5th metacarpal bones on the dorsum of the wrist, traverses the forearm beween the ulna and radius, and continues upward across the olecranon and the lateral aspects of the upper arm to the shoulder. Here it intersects the Small Intestine channel at point **SI 12** (*Bing Feng*) and meets the Governing channel at point **Du 14** (*Da Zhui*) before crossing back over the shoulder. It then intersects the Gall Bladder channel at point **GB 21** (*Jian Jing*), from which it enters the supraclavicular fossa and travels to the mid-chest region at point **Ren 17** (*Shan Zhong*). From here, the channel joins with the Pericardium and descends across the **diaphragm** to the abdomen linking successively with the upper, middle and lower burners of the Triple Burner, to which this channel belongs.

A **branch** of the main channel separates in the chest at point **Ren 17** (*Shan Zhong*) and ascends to emerge superficially from the supraclavicular fossa at the neck. Here, it proceeds upward behind the ear, intersecting the Gall Bladder channel at points **GB 6** (*Xuan Li*) and **GB 4** (*Han Yan*) on the forehead before winding downward across the cheek to below the **eye**. It intersects the Small Intestine channel at point **SI 18** (*Quan Liao*).

Another **branch** separates behind the auricle and enters the ear. It then emerges in front of the ear where it intersects the Small Intestine channel at point **SI 19** (*Ting Gong*), crosses in front of the Gall Bladder channel at point **GB 3** (*Shang Guan*) and traverses the cheek to terminate at the outer cantus at point **SJ 23** (*Si Zhu Kong*).

Chapter 4 of the *Ling Shu* states that the Triple Burner channel connects with its Lower Uniting (Lower *He* Sea) point, **UB 39** (*Wei Yang*). Chapter 2 adds that this branch fo the Triple Burner channel emerges from UB 39 and follows the course of the Bladder channel to join with the Bladder

San Jiao Channel Sx: swelling and pain in the throat, pain in the cheek and jaw, redness in the eyes, deafness, pain behind the ear or along the lateral aspect of the shoulder and upper arm.

San Jiao Organ Sx: abdominal distension, hardness and fullness in the lower abdomen, enuresis, frequent urination, edema, dysuresis.

*Image from CAM, description from ACT

Xi **Cleft**

Site where qi and blood of the channel are deeply converged

12 regular and 4 extras have Xi cleft

Indications: 1.

2.

3.

Lu___ St___ Ht___ UB___ P____ GB___

LI___ Sp__ SI___ K____ SJ____ Liv____

1. **Pain and numbness of the knee, gastric pain, mastitis,** motor impairment of the lower extremities:

2. Cardiac pain, palpitation, epistaxis, hematemesis, hemoptysis, chest pain, furuncle, epilepsy:

3. Headache, swelling of the face, sore throat, borborygmus, abdominal pain, aching of the shoulder and arm:

4. **Blurring of vision, pain in the shoulder**, elbow and arm:

5. Abdominal pain and distension, diarrhea, edema, dysuria, nocturnal emission, irregular menstruation, dysmenorrhea:

6., Abdominal pain, hypochondriac pain, diarrhea, **hernia**, uterine bleeding, prolonged lochia:

7. Mania, epilepsy, infantile convulsion, **backache,** pain in the external malleolus, motor impairment and pain of the lower extremities:

8. Amenorrhea, irregular menstruation, dysmenorrhea, prolapse of uterus, dysuria, blurring of vision:

9. Cardiac pain, hysteria, **night sweating**, hemoptysis, epsitaxis, sudden loss of voice:

10. *Cough, pain in the chest, asthma, hemoptysis, sore throat, spasmodic pain of the elbow and arm:*

11. *Deafness, pain in the ear, epilepsy, pain of the arm:*

12. Pain in the neck, chest, thigh and hypochondriac region, rabies:

Confluent Points (review)   *Xi Cleft (4 of the 8 Extraordinary Channels)*
Yin Wei confluent: *Yin Wei Xi Cleft:*
Yang Wei confluent: *Yang Wei Xi Cleft:*
Yin Qiao confluent: *Yin Qiao Xi Cleft:*
Yang Qiao confluent: *Yang Qiao Xi Cleft:*

(CAM indications do not really match channel symptoms, so they are not included here)

Yuan _Source_

Yuan qi originates below the umbilicus btw kidneys, disperses to zang fu to limbs via_____.
Yuan points is where yuan qi is retained,. They treat disorders of_____(which organs).
(On the Yin channels, the _Yuan_ Pt=_Shu_ Stream Pt)

Lu___	St___	Ht___	UB___	P____	GB____
LI___	Sp___	SI___	K____	SJ____	Liv____

1. Cardiac pain, palpitation, stomachache, vomiting, mental disorders, epilepsy, stuffy chest, pain in the hypochondriac region, convulsion, insomnia, irritability, foul breath:

2. Pain in the neck, swelling in the axillary region, pain in the hypochondriac region, vomiting, acid regurgitation, muscular atrophy of the lower limbs, pain and swelling of the external malleolus, malaria:

3. Pain in the arm, shoulder and wrist, malaria, deafness, thirst:
(direct moxa to regulate women's hormones/menses)

4. Headache, dizziness and vertigo, insomnia, congestion, swelling and pain of the eye, depression, infantile convulsion, **deviation of the mouth,** pain in the hypochondriac region, uterine bleeding, **hernia,** enuresis, retention of urine, epilepsy, pain in the anterior aspect of the medial malleolus:

5. Gastric pain, abdominal distension, constipation, dysentery, vomiting, diarrhea, borborygmus, sluggishness, beriberi:

6. Febrile diseases with anhidrosis, headache, rigidity of the neck, contracture of the fingers, pain in the wrist, jaundice:

7. Cough, asthma, hemoptysis, sore throat, palpitation, pain in the chest, wrist and arm:
(avoid puncturing: _____)

8. Headache, pain in the neck, redness, swelling and pain of the eye, epistaxis, nasal obstruction, rhinorrhea, toothache, deafness, swelling of the face, sore throat, parotitis, trismus, **facial paralysis, febrile disease with anhidrosis, hidrosis**, abdominal pain, dysentery, constipation, amenorrhea, **delayed labour**, infantile convulsion, pain, weakness and motor impairment of the upper limb:
(trismus: lockjaw)

9. Cardiac pain, irritability, palpitation, hysteria, amnesia, **insomnia**, mania, epilepsy, dementia, pain in the hypochondriac region, feverish sensation in the palm, yellowish sclera:

10. Pain of the upper teeth, redness and swelling of the dorsum of the foot, facial paralysis, muscular atrophy and motor impairment of the foot:
(Avoid puncturing:_____)

11. Headache, neck rigidity, pain in the lower back and thigh, epilepsy:

12. Sore throat, toothache, deafness, tinnitus, dizziness, spitting of blood, asthma, thirst, irregular menstruation, insomnia, nocturnal emission, impotence, frequency of micturition*, pain in the lower back:

*micturition: urination

Superficial (*fŭ mai i*浮脈)
Can be felt easily with gentle touch.
Indicates:

Deep (*chén mai* 沉脈)
Felt only on heavy pressure.
Indicates:
Deep & forceful indicates:
Deep & weak indicates:

Slow (*chí mai* 遲脈)
Less than 4 beats per breath (<60 beats/sec)
Indicates:
Slow & forceful, indicates:
Slow & weak indicates:

Rapid (*shuò mai* 數脈)
More than 5 beats per breath (>90 beats/sec)
Indicates:
Rapid Forceful:
Rapid weak:

Deficient (*xū mai* 虛脈)
Forceless on all three regions at all three levels
Indicates:

Excess (*shí mai* 實脈)
Forceful pulse on all three regions at all three levels
Indicates:

– – – – – – – – – – – – – – – – – – –

Surging/Flooding (*hóng mai* 洪脈)
Broad, large and forceful like roaring
waves which come on powerfully
and fade away
Indicates:
If surging pulse lacks the momentum of
roaring waves it is called a "large pulse"

Tense/Tight (*jĭn mai* 緊脈)
Tight and forceful, like a stretched rope
Indicates: 1.
            2.
            3.

Soft (*rú mai* 濡脈)
Superficial & thready, hits without strength
Indicates:

Thready (*xì mai* 細脈)
Like a fine thread, distinct and clear
Indicates:

Weak (*ruò mai* 弱脈)
Deep & thready, hits without strength
Indicates:

Rolling/Slippery (*huá mai* 滑脈)
Smooth & flowing, like pearls rolling on a dish.
Indicates 1.
            2.
            3.
(This pulse is normal for:)

Abrupt (*cù mai* 促脈)
Hurried & rapid, with irregularly missed beats
Indicates 1.
            2.
            3.

Hesitant/Choppy (*sè mai* 澀脈)
Rough and uneven.
Choppy forceful: 1.
                  2.
(less commonly Choppy weak)
1.   2.

Knotted (*jié mai* 結脈)
Slow, with irregularly missed beats
Indicates: 1.
           2.
           3.
           4.

Regularly Intermittent (*dài mai* 代脈)
Slow & weak, with regularly missed beats
Associated with decline of *Zang* Qi
Also indicates:

String-taut/Bowstring (*xián mai* 弦脈)
Taut, straight and long, like a violin string
Indicates: 1.
            2.
            3.

Qi & Blood Pathology

Qi Syndromes:
Four main categories of Qi imbalance:
<u>two deficiency</u>
1.
2.
<u>two excess</u>
3.
4.

1. Sx: dizziness, blurred vision, dislike of speaking, lassitude, **spontaneous sweating, all worse on exertion**
T: pale
P: deficient
Dx:
Etiology: often due to weakness after long illness, feebleness in old age, improper diet, or excess of strain or stress.

2. Sx: dizziness, blurred vision, lassitude, bearing down distending sensation in the abdominal region, prolapse of anus or uterus, gastroptosis, renal ptosis
T: pale
P: deficient
Dx:
(a subcategory of Qi Deficiency)
Etiology: same as Qi Deficiency

3. Sx: distension & pain
(distension more severe than pain, both wax and wane with no fixed position,
onset often related to emotions, sx may be alleviated temporarily by belching or flatus)
Dx:
Etiology: mental depression, improper diet, exogenous pathogen, sprain, or contusion.

4. Rebellious Qi (affects mainly 3 organs):
Rebellious Lung Qi Sx:
Etiology: External pathogen or Phlegm Retention in Lung (Fails to D&D)

Rebellious Stomach Qi Sx:
Etiology: Retention of fluid, phlegm or Food, or External pathogen

Excessive ascendant Liver Qi Sx:
Etiology: Injury of the Liver by anger, upward disturbance of Qi, then of Qi & Fire

Blood Syndromes:
1. Sx: pale or sallow complexion, pale lips, dizziness, blurred vision, palpitations, insomnia, numb hands & feet
T: pale
P: thready
Dx:
Etiology:

2. Sx: pain, mass, tumors, hemorrhage, ecchymosis or petechiae*
(petchiae: small purplish hemorrhagic spots on the skin that occur in patients with platelet deficiencies (thrombocytopenia) and in many febrile illnesses)
T: purplish
P: choppy
Dx:
Etiology (many causes):

3. Sx: mental restlessness, or mania in severe cases, dry mouth with no desire to drink, possible various hemorrhagic syndromes, profuse menstrual flow in women
Dx:
T: deep red
P: rapid
Etiology: often due to invasion of External Heat or obstruction of Liver Qi turning to fire.

Precious Supplementary Prescriptions states that "All diseases start from stagnation of qi and blood. Needling may promote smooth circulation of qi and blood…"

Other Causes of Disease
-Weak constitution
-Over-exertion (mental or physical overwork)
-Excessive sexual activity
-Diet (malnutrition, overeating, cold/raw, sweet, greasy & fried, hot, spicy)
(Do not eat in a hurry, discussing work while eating, going straight back to work
after eating, eating too late in the evening, in a state of emotional tension.)
-Trauma
-Parasites & poisons
-Wrong treatment (Iatrogenic)
Also: 7 Emotions (七情)

REGULATE QI

herb (yao 藥)	flavor (wei 味)		temp (qi 氣)	channels								
Chen Pi	acrid, bitter	aromatic	warm	Lu	Sp	St						
Ju Hong	acrid, bitter	aromatic	warm	Lu		St						
Qing Pi	bitter, acrid		warm			St	GB	Liv				
Da Fu Pi	acrid		sl. warm		Sp	St			LI	SI		
Zhi Shi	bitter, acrid		sl. cold		Sp	St			LI			
Xiang Fu	acrid, sl. bitter, sl. sweet		neutral					Liv		SJ		
Mu Xiang	acrid, bitter		warm		Sp	St	GB		LI			
Wu Yao	acrid		warm	Lu	Sp						UB	K
Chen Xiang	acrid, bitter	aromatic	warm		Sp	St						K
Tan Xiang	acrid	aromatic	warm	Lu	Sp	St						
Xie Bai	acrid, bitter		warm	Lu		St			LI			
Fo Shou	acrid, bitter		sl. warm	Lu	Sp	St		Liv				
Mei Gui Hua	sweet, sl. bitter		warm		Sp			Liv				
Chuan Lian Zi	bitter	sl. toxic	cold			St		Liv		SI	UB	
Shi Di	bitter, astringent		neutral	Lu		St						

FOOD STAGNATION

herb (yao 藥)	flavor (wei 味)		temp (qi 氣)	channels				
Shan Zha	sour, sweet		sl. warm	Liv	Sp	St		
Mai Ya (barley)	sweet		neutral	Liv	Sp	St		
Gu Ya (rice)	sweet		neutral		Sp	St		
Shen Qu	sweet, acrid		warm		Sp	St		
Ji Nei Jin	sweet		neutral		Sp	St	UB	SI
Lai Fu Zi	acrid, sweet		neutral		Sp	St		Lu

Herbs
Regulate Qi

Chen Pi	*Qing Pi*	*Mu Xiang*	*Fo Shou*
Ju Hong	*Da Fu Pi*	*Wu Yao*	*Mei Gui Hua*
Ju Ye	*Zhi Shi*	*Chen Xiang*	*Chuan Lian Zi*
Ju Luo	*Zhi Ke*	*Tan Xiang*	*Shi Di*
Ju He	*Xiang Fu*	*Xie Bai*	

Questions 1- 6 are all part of *citrus reticulata* (tangerine).

1. _____ , the ripened peel, enters the Lung, Spleen & Stomach. It **regulates Qi, improves the transporting function of the Spleen, dries Damp & transforms phlegm**, and is used with tonifying herbs to prevent their cloying nature from causing stagnation.

2. _____ , the zest, is acrid, bitter and warm and enters the Lung and Stomach channels. It is more drying and aromatic than *Chen Pi,*, but is less effective in harmonizing the middle and regulating the Middle. Originally, this was the herb in *Er Chen Tang*, though *Chen Pi* is often substituted.

3. _____ , the unripened peel, is green and so it enters the Liver & GB channels (as well as Stomach) to **spread Liver Qi and break up stagnant Qi in the chest, breast or hypochondirac region.** It also dissipates clumps, reduces food stagnation, dries Damp and transforms Phlegm (it is more like *Ju Hong*)

4. _____ , the seed, treats "seed" shaped problems such as nodules, hernia, breast lumps, swollen lymph nodes and fibroids (Dampness congesting into phlegm nodules).

5. _____ , the white pith on the inside of the peel, moves Qi and transforms phlegm to treat cough and wheezing. It also opens the meridians.

6. _____ , the leaf, is green to smooth Liver Qi. It treats pain in the hypochondrium, mastitis, breast abscess, lumps and tumors.

7. _____ is the **Imperial herb to regulate menstruation** and alleviate pain, for irregular menstruation **due to constrained Liver Qi**. (The other Imperial herb for Irregular menses and pain due to Blood deficiency or Blood stasis is Dang Gui). It is acrid, slightly bitter, slightly sweet and neutral. It enters the Liver and the San Jiao. (Dr. Shen liked to use a small dose of 1.5 qian to treat the Heart)

Both of the following herbs come from *citrus aurantium* (bitter orange).

8. _____ has a **stronger action,** breaks up Qi stagnation and reduces accumulations. It descends downward, mostly used for **unblocking the obstruction of bowel movements.**

9. _____ has a **milder action**, moves Qi and reduces distention. It is used mostly for **distention and fullness of the epigastrium and abdomen.**

10. _____ moves Qi downward to reduce stagnation, and **promotes urination to reduce superficial edema.**

11. _____ **stops hiccups.**

12. Bitter, cold, and slightly toxic, _____ effectively spreads Liver Qi and alleviates pain, often used in **Liver constraint with Heat signs, and can also kill parasites.**

13. Yet another Qi regulating citrus fruit, _____ gently spreads and regulates Liver Qi, mildly dries Damp and transforms phlegm, and harmonizes the Stomach and strengthens the Spleen.

14. _____ moves Qi, alleviates pain, **warms and unblocks the channels**, and **warms the Kidneys** for frequent urination or incontinence.

15. _____, moves Qi, descends rebellious Qi (for excess or deficient wheezing, vomiting or belching from Middle jiao deficient Cold) and aids the Kidneys in grasping Qi. This expensive aged wood should never be decocted, but dissolved in the finished liquid.

16. _____ moves Qi and alleviates pain. This tree takes 50-70 years to mature, and is necessarily cut down (not simply pruned) as we use the heartwood for medicinal and perfume purposes.

17. _____ is acrid and warm to **move Qi** and disperse, aromatic to **revive the Spleen**. It effectively moves Stomach and Intestine Qi to reduce distension and alleviate pain. It is also **combined with Qi tonics to prevent Qi stagnation** (as in *Gui Pi Tang*)

Food Stagnation

Shan Zha	*Shen Qu*
Gu Ya	*Ji Nei Jin*
Mai Ya	*Lai Fu Zi*

1. _____ & _____ are most important for treating food stagnation from grains.

2. _____ is best for over indulgence in meat. Additionally, in Western herbology, its Western counterpart is used to strengthen the Heart and arterial walls and clean the blood.

3. _____ is best for problems related to overindulgence in alcohol and starchy foods. It harmonizes the Middle Jiao.

4. _____ strongly reduces food stagnation.
With *Sang Piao Xiao, Long Gu,* and *Mu Li* to secure essence and stop bedwetting.
With *Jian Qian Cao* to dissolves stones (urinary or biliary tract, therefore enters the UB & GB channels)

5. _____ most strongly descends Qi and reduces phlegm. It is the only herb in this category that enters the Lung channel. (most effective with Excess conditions).

DUI YAO
Synergistic Herb Combinations

Chen Pi & Sang Bai Pi
One transforms and prevents the production of phlegm
The other drains and clears the Lungs
Together they effectively **clear the Lungs, transform phlegm,**
Rectify the Qi, **stop coughing and calm Asthma**
    Wu Pi San

Sang Bai Pi & Sheng Jiang Pi
One promotes urination by descending Lung Qi and opening the water pathways
The other transforms Damp and disperses edema.
Together, through dispersing and descending,
they restore the Lung's role in water metabolism
To facilitate the smooth flow of fluids into the UB.
    Wu Pi San

Fu Ling & Gui Zhi
Together they warm & transform water & fluids,
Unblock the Yang, and promote urination.
    Wu Ling San

(Han) Fang Ji & Huang Qi
One drains and descends.
The other supplements and raises.
Together they **support the *Zheng Qi***
& drain *Xie Qi* at the same time,
regulate Qi mechanism of ascending & descending,
and **strongly promote urination**.
    Fang Ji Huang Qi Tang
Fang Ji promotes urination by draining the UB
Huang Qi promotes urination by supplementing Lung Qi for descending & dispersing
+ *Bai Zhu* which promotes urination by fortifying the Spleen Qi to transform Damp,

Chen Pi & Hou Po
Chen Pi regulates the Qi, thereby transforming Damp
Hou Po dispels Damp and disperses fullness.
Together they revive the Spleen and improve appetite.
    Ping Wei San
    Huo Xiang Zheng Qi San

Formulas
Expel Damp

Wu Ling San
Zhu Ling Tang
Wu Pi San
Fang Ji Huang Qi Tang
Ping Wei San

Bu Huan Jin Zheng Qi San
Huo Xiang Zheng Qi San
Yin Chen Hao Tang
Ba Zheng San
Shao Yao Tang

Zhen Wu Tang
Bi Xie Fen Qing Yin
Du Huo Ji Sheng Tang

Promote Urination & Leach out Damp
1. Action: resolves Damp, reduces edema, regulates qi, strengthens the Spleen
Skin edema (pi shui) due to:
    1. Wind invasion disrupting the Lung's D&D fxn
    2. Kidney Yang deficiency leading to fluid/Damp accumulation
    3. Spleen deficiency with vigorous Damp & Qi stagnation
Formula:

2. Feng Shui (wind edema) due to external deficiency with Wind Damp invasion.
Formula:

3. Action: Promote urination, clear Heat, nourish Yin
Injury from Cold entering Yang Ming or Shao Yin where it transforms to Heat.
(This formula promotes urination without injuring the Yin, and stabilizes the Yin without causing retention of pathogen, largely due to e jiao)
Formula:

4. Action: Promote urination, drain Damp, strengthen the Spleen, warm the Yang, & promote the transforming functions of Qi.
Three etiologies:
    1. Water buildup from Tai Yang External disorder penetrating the UB (Tai Yang organ)
    2. Spleen deficiency with internal Damp & water accumulation
    3. Retention of congested fluids in the lower burner (Tan Yin)
Formula:

Transform Damp Turbidity
5. External Wind Cold with concurrent Internal Cold Damp stagnation:

6. Damp Cold stagnating in the Spleen & Stomach:

7. Ping Wei San + Huo Xiang, Ban Xia
Externally contracted sudden turmoil disorder, stronger ability to transform turbid Damp and regulate Qi:

Clear Damp Heat
8. Hot or Bloody painful urinary dysfunction due to Damp Heat clumping in the lower jiao:

9. Damp Heat lodged in the Intestines, causing Qi & Blood stagnation:

10. Yang Type Damp Heat jaundice:

Warm & Transform Damp
11. Cloudy painful urinary dysfunction (gao lin) due to def Cold in the lower Jiao:

12. Kidney Yang deficiency, or Spleen & Kidney Yang deficiency, with retention of pathogenic water: (Also for External Tai Yang W/C)

Dispel Wind Damp
13. Painful obstruction with Liver & Kidney deficiency (W/C/D Bi):

Du Huo Ji Sheng Tang
4 to expel W/D/C from bones, sinews, & channels
1.
2.
3.
4.
4 to expel W/D & tonify Kidney & Liver
5.
6.
7.
8.
Si Wu Tang
9.
10.
11.
12.
Si Jun Zi Tang (-Bai Zhu)
13.
14.
15.

Ping Wei San
1.
2.
3.
Plus 3 amigos (_zhi gan cao_)

Wu Ling San and _Zhu Ling Tang_ both promote urination and drain Damp.
Both formulas have (which herbs):
1.
2.
3.
Wu Ling San (Drains Vigorous Damp)
is for when the disease is still active in the exterior, and focuses on unblocking the flow of Yang to encourage the transformation of Qi.
The two additional herbs are:
4.
5.
Zhu Ling Tang (Drains Vigorous Heat)
treats pathogens which have transformed into Internal Heat, by clearing Heat and nourishing Yin. The two additional herbs are:
4.
5.

Wu Pi San
Lungs (D&D fxn of Lung to restore water metab., facilitate the smooth flow of fluid to UB)
1.
2.
Spleen (leaches out Damp, promotes urination, strengthens Spleen):
3.
Move Qi, eliminate Qi stagnation:
4.
5.

Ba Zheng San vs. _Dao Chi San_

Ba Zheng San strongly unblocks painful urinary dysfunction, does not nourish the Yin at all, and focuses on the lower burner symptoms (urinary retention with lower abdominal distension and pain)

Dao Chi San focuses on the upper jiao (irritability and mouth sores), nourishes the Yin, but has much weaker effect on painful urinary dysfunction.

Gall Bladder – Foot *Shao Yang*

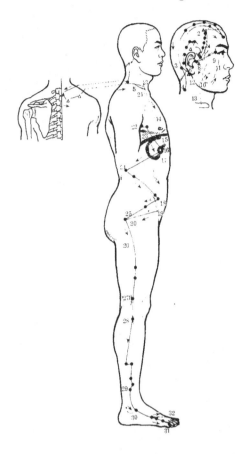

Originates:

Connects with
  Organs:
  Structures:

Xi: *Jing* Well:
Luo: *Ying* Spring:
Yuan: *Shu* Stream:
               Jing River:
Front *Mu:*   *He* Sea
Back *Shu:*

Influential Point:
  of :

Influential Point:
  of:

Confluent Pt (8 extras):
  of which channel:

Crossing Points:

Channel Pathway
This channel begins at the **outer canthus** of the **eye** and traverses the temple to **SJ 22** *(He Liao)*. It then ascends to the corner of the forehead where it intersects **St 8** *(Tou Wei)* before descending behind the ear. From here, it proceeds along the neck in front of the San Jiao channel, crosses the Small Intestine channel at **SI 17** *(Tian Rong)*, then, at the top of the shoulder, turns back and runs behind the San Jiao channel to intersect the Du channel at **Du 14** *(Da Zhui)* on the spine. Finally, the channel turns downward into the supraclvicular fossa.
One branch of the main channel emerges behind the auricle and enters the **ear** at **SJ 17** *(Yi Feng)*. Emerging in front of the ear, this branch intersect the Small Intestine channel at **SI 19** *(Ting Gong)*, and the Stomach channel at **St 7** *(Xiang Guan)*, before terminating behind the **outer canthus.**
Another branch separates at the outer and proceds downward to point **St 5** *(Da Ying)* on the jaw. Then, crossing the San Jiao channel, it returns upward to the infraorbital region before descednign again ot the neck, where it joins the original channel in the supraclavicular fossa. From here it descends further into the chest, crossing the diaphragm and connecting with the **Liver**, before joining its associated Organ, the **Gall Bladder**. Continuing along the **inside of the ribs**, it emerges in the inguinal region of the lower abdomen and winds around the genitals, submerging again in the hip at point GB 30 *(Huan Tiao)*.
Yet another vertical branch runs downward from the supraclavicular fossa to the axilla and the lateral aspect of the chest. It crosses the ribs and intersects the Liver channel at point **Liv 13** *(Zhang Men)* before turning back to the sacral region, where it crosses the Bladder channel at **UB 31** *(Shang Liao)* **to UB 34** *(Xia Liao)*. This branch then descends ot the hip joint and continues down the lateral side of the thigh and knee, passing along the anterior aspect of the fibula to its lower end. Here it crosses in front of the lateral malleolus and traverses the dorsum of the foot, entering the seam between the 4th and 5th metatarsal bones before terminating at the lateral side of the tip of the 4th toe at GB 44 *(Zu Qiao Yin)*.
Finally, a **branch** separtes on the dorsum of the foot at point GB 41 *(Lin Qi)* and runs between the 1st and 2nd metatarsal bones to the medial tip of the big toe, then crosses under the toenail to join with the Liver channel at point **Liv 1** *(Da Dun)*.

Gall Bladder Channel Sx: alternating fever and chills, headache, ashen complexion; pain in the eye or jaw, swelling in the sub-axillary region, scrofula, deafness, pain along the channel in the hip region, leg or foot.

Gall Bladder Organ Sx: pain in the ribs, vomiting, bitter taste in the mouth, chest pain.

Liver- Foot *Jue Yin*

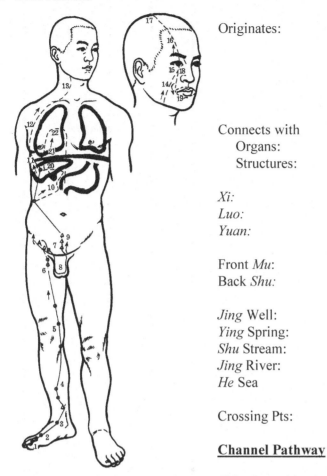

Fig. 16 The Liver Meridian of Foot-Jueyin

Originates:

Connects with
  Organs:
    Structures:

Xi:
Luo:
Yuan:

Front *Mu*:
Back *Shu:*

Jing Well:
Ying Spring:
Shu Stream:
Jing River:
He Sea

Crossing Pts:

Channel Pathway

This channel begins on the dorsum of the big toe, continues across the foot to a point one unit in front of the medial malleolus, and proceeds upward to point **Sp 6** *(San Yin Jiao)* where it intersects the Spleen channel. From here, it continues up the medial aspect of the lower leg, re-crossing the Spleen channel *eight units above the medial malleolus*, and thereafter running posterior to that channel over the knee and thigh. Winding around the **genitals,** the channel eneters the lower abdomen where it meets the Ren channel at points **Ren 2** *(Qu Gu)*, **Ren 3** *(Zhong Ji)*, and **Ren 4** *(Guan Yuan)* before skirting the Stomach channel and joining with its associated organ, the **Liver**, and connecting with the **Gall Bladder**. Then the channel continues upward across the diaphragm and costal region, traverses the neck posterior to the pharynx, and enters the nasopharynx, connecting with the **tissue surrounding the eye**. Finally, the channel ascends across the forehead and meets the Du channel at the **vertex**.

    A branch separates below the eye and encircles the **inside of the lips**.

    Another branch separates in the Liver, crosses the diaphragm and reaches the **Lung**.

Liver Channel Sx: headache, vertigo, blurred vision, tinnitus, fever, spasms in the extremities.

Liver Organ Sx: fullness or pain in the costal region or chest, hard lumps in the upper abdomen, abdominal pain, vomiting, jaundice, loose stool, pain in the lower abdomen, hernia, enuresis, retention of urine, dark urine.

*Image from CAM, description from ACT

LIVER & GALLBLADDER SYNDROMES

	Tongue	Pulse	Palpitations	Breathing	Sweating	Insomnia	Sleep	Dream Disturbed Sleep	Poor Memory	Other Sx
Liver Qi Stagnation										
Liver Fire										
Liver Yang Rising										
Internal Liver Wind										
Wind due to: Yang Rising										
Wind due to: Extreme Heat										
Wind due to: Blood Deficiency	For clinical manifestations see Liver Blood Deficiency below									
Liver Blood Deficiency										
Liver Channel Cold										
Liver GB Damp Heat										
Damp Heat in Liver Channel	Distinguishing Sx: Eczema of scrotum, swelling / burning pain of testes, yellow / foul smelling leukorrhea, pruritis vulvae									

Du

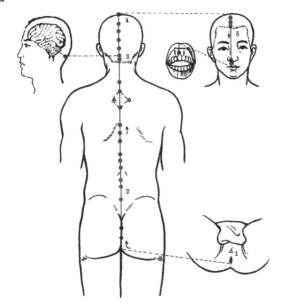

Fig. 17 The Governor Vessel

Sea of:

Confluent Point:

Paired with:

Luo:

Crossing Points:

Du Channel Sx: Stiffness & pain along the spine, heavy sensation in the head, vertigo, shaking, mental disorders, febrile disease, Qi rushing toward the heart, colic, constipation, enuresis, hemorrhoids & infertility

Ren

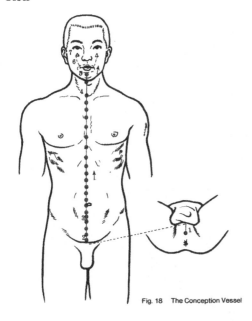

Fig. 18 The Conception Vessel

Sea of:

Confluent Point:

Paired with:

Luo:

Crossing Points:

Ren Channel Sx: pathological symptoms in the Yin channels, esp associated with Liver & Kidneys, closely related to pregnancy, infertility and other urogenital problems, leukorrhea, irregular menstruation, colic.

Images from CAM, descriptions from ACT

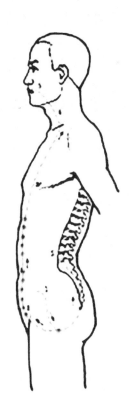

Chong

 Sea of:

Confluent Point:

Paired with:

Crossing Points:

Chong Channel Sx: gynecological disorders, male sexual irregularities including impotence, abdominal pain or colic.

Dai Channel

Confluent Point:

Paired with:

      Crossing Points:

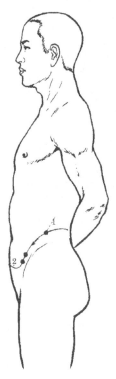

Fig. 20   The Belt Vessel

Theory & Diagnosis

Tongue

Coating
Thin indicates: normal or if pathological, then:
Thick:
Greasy:
Thin, white:
Thin Yellow:
Thick, greasy, yellow:
Scanty, less coat:

Body
Pale, dry:
Pale, wet:
Red without coating:
Reddish purple:
Bluish purple:
Distended dark veins under the tongue:

Shape
Swollen edges, scalloped:
Thin, pale:
Thin, red:
Deviated:
Sore covered:

Eight Treatment Methods (Herbal)

1.Method:_____   5. Method:_____

Application:_____   Application:_____

2. Method:_____   6. Method:_____

Application:_____   Application:_____

3. Method:_____   7. Method:_____

Application:_____   Application:_____

4. Method:_____   8. Method:_____

Application:_____   Application:_____

STOP BLEEDING

herb (yao 藥)	flavor (wei 味)		temp (qi 氣)	Liv	Ht	Sp	Lu	St	LI	K	SI	UB
pu huang	sweet, acrid		neutral	**Liv**	Ht	Sp						
xian he cao	**bitter**, acrid		neutral	**Liv**		Sp	Lu					
san qi	sweet, sl. bitter		warm	**Liv**				St	LI			
bai ji	**bitter**, sweet		cool	**Liv**			Lu	St				
da ji	sweet		cool	**Liv**		Sp						
di yu	**bitter**, sour		sl. cold	**Liv**				St	LI			
huai hua mi	**bitter**		cool	**Liv**					LI			
qian cao gen	**bitter**		cold	**Liv**	Ht							
ce bai ye	**bitter**	astringent	sl. cold	**Liv**	Ht				LI			
ai ye	**bitter**, acrid		warm	**Liv**		Sp				K		
ou jie	sweet	astringent	neutral	**Liv**			Lu	St				
bai mao gen	sweet		cold				Lu	St			SI	UB

INVIGORATE BLOOD

herb (yao 藥)	flavor (wei 味)		temp (qi 氣)	Liv	GB	Pc	Ht	Sp	St	Lu	LI	UB	K
chuan xiong	**acrid**		warm	**Liv**	GB	Pc							
dan shen	**bitter**		sl. cold	**Liv**		Pc	**Ht**						
ji xue teng	**bitter**, sweet		warm	**Liv**			**Ht**	Sp					
yan hu suo	**acrid, bitter**		warm	**Liv**			**Ht**		St	Lu			
yu jin	**acrid, bitter**		cool	**Liv**			**Ht**			Lu			
jiang huang	**acrid, bitter**		warm	**Liv**				Sp	St				
yi mu cao	**acrid, bitter**		sl. cold	**Liv**			**Ht**					UB	
ze lan	**bitter, acrid**	aromatic	sl. warm	**Liv**				Sp					
si gua luo	sweet		neutral	**Liv**					St	Lu			
chi shao	sour, **bitter**		sl. cold	**Liv**				Sp					
tao ren	**bitter**, sweet		neutral	**Liv**			**Ht**			Lu	LI		
hong hua	**acrid**		warm	**Liv**			**Ht**						
e zhu	**bitter, acrid**		warm	**Liv**				Sp					
san leng	**bitter, acrid**		neutral	**Liv**				Sp					
ru xiang	**acrid, bitter**		warm	**Liv**			**Ht**	Sp					
mo yao	**bitter**		neutral	**Liv**			**Ht**	Sp					
niu xi	**bitter**, sour		neutral	**Liv**									K
wang bu liu xing	**bitter**		neutral	**Liv**					St				
zi ran tong	**acrid, bitter**		neutral	**Liv**									K
su mu	sweet, salty		neutral	**Liv**			**Ht**	Sp					
wu ling zhi	**bitter**, sweet		warm	**Liv**				Sp					
chuan shan jia	salty		cool	**Liv**					St				
shui zhi	salty, **bitter**	sl. toxic	neutral	**Liv**								UB	
tu bie chong	salty	toxic	cold	**Liv**			**Ht**	Sp					

Herbs

Stop Bleeding

Pu Huang	**Da Ji**	**Ce Bai Ye**
Xian He Cao	*Di Yu*	*Ai Ye*
San Qi	*Huai Hua Mi*	*Ou Jie*
Bai Ji	*Qian Cao Gen*	*Bai Mao Gen*

These herbs stop bleeding in different ways: by <u>cooling</u>, <u>astringing</u>, <u>invigorating</u> or <u>warming</u>. As bleeding is the branch, it is important to combine them with herbs that address the root (such as Clear Heat, Cool Blood, or Tonify Qi, Warm Yang etc.)

1. _____ **warms the womb,** pacifies the fetus, and disperses cold to alleviate pain. It is especially good for **gynecological disorders.**

2. Sweet, slightly bitter, and warm, _____ **stops bleeding and transforms Blood Stasis.** It is the **Imperial hemostatic herb** for most types of bleeding and for traumatic injuries with hematoma, swelling and pain. Also, it is the main ingredient of *Yunnan Baiyao.*

3. Sweet, acrid and neutral, _____ **stops bleeding** (from external injury or internal bleeding), **invigorates the Blood and dispels stasis.**

4. Bitter, acrid and neutral, _____**stops bleeding from either Cold or Heat, Excess or Deficiency.** Additionally it **alleviates diarrhea** and **kills parasites.**

5. Often used for **hematuria during Heat type Painful *Lin* syndrome,** _____ clears Heat and promotes urination. It cools the Blood and clears Heat from the Stomach and Lungs (for nose bleeds or coughing of Blood).

6. _____ enters the **Large Intestine. and Liver channels**, and is especially important for **bleeding hemorrhoids**, and treats red eyes and dizziness due to Liver Heat.

7. Sweet, astringent and neutral, _____ is relatively mild and is therefore used as an auxiliary herb to stop bleeding, for various types (especially hematemesis and hemoptysis). Raw to invigorate blood and stop bleeding, charred to astringe to stop bleeding. This herb is used in food.

8. _____ & _____ cools the Blood, **stops bleeding (especially in urine or stool), reduces swelling and generates flesh (for sores).**

9. _____ restrains leakage of Blood and stops bleeding, mainly from the Lungs and Stomach. It also reduces swelling and generates flesh. (Dr Fu taught that it kills *Zhai Chong*, TB)

10. Bitter and Cold, enters the Heart and Liver, _____, cools the Blood to stop bleeding and invigorates the Blood to dispel stasis.

11. _____ **cools Blood to stop bleeding,** stops coughing and expels phlegm, **and heals burns (topically)**

Invigorate Blood

Chuan Xiong   Yi Mu Cao   E Zhu   Zi Ran Tong
Dan Shen   Ze Lan   San Leng   Su Mu
Ji Xue Teng   Wu Ling Zhi   Ru Xiang   Chuan Shan Zha (endangered)
Yan Hu Suo   Chi Shao   Mo Yao   Shui Zhi
Yu Jin   Tao Ren   Niu Xi   Tu Bie Chong
Jiang Huang   Hong Hua   Wang Bu Liu Xing

1. _____ is similar (though cooler temperature) to the formula *Si Wu Tang*, in that it **both moves & nourishes** the Blood. It is bitter and slightly cold, enters the Heart, Pc, and Liver. It invigorates the Blood, breatks up Blood stasis, especially in the lower abdomen, and clears heat to soothe irritability.

2. _____ is powerful for breaking up Blood stasis. It also **moistens the intestines** and unblock sthe bowel.

3. Primarily used for gynecological patterns of Blood stasis, _____ is frequently combined with *Tao Ren*. It enterst eh Heart and Liver, and is acrid and warm.

4. _____ **guides blood downward** as well as **nourishing the Liver and Kidney** to strengthen the sinews and bones. (Its Sichuan counterpart is stronger at invigorating the Blood and promoting urination)

5._____ invigorates the Blood, moves Qi and alleviates pain. It is recognized as an **effective analgesic** for Qi and Blood stagnation anywhere in the Body.

6. _____ is **primarily used for gynecological disorders** due to Blood stasis. It is acrid, bitter, slightly cold and enters the Heart, Liver and UB. Additionally it **promotes urination** (translates to "benefit mother herb")

7. **Often combined for traumatic injuries, internally and/or topically,** _____ & _____ invigorate Blood, move Qi and alleviate pain.

8. _____ is Cold in nature, clears Blood Heat. (Some texts put it in the category of "Clear Heat, Cool Blood")

9. _____ & _____ are known for **breaking up Blood stasis,** and are often combined for severe accumulations such as masses.

10. _____ is recognized as the "Qi herb in the Blood level" as it moves both Blood and Qi. It also **expels wind and alleviates pain.** It is the **Imperial herb for headaches.**

11. _____ invigorates Blood (raw), alleviates pain, and stops bleeding (charred).

12. _____ moves both Qi and Blood, enters the **Liver** to affect the chest and hypochondrium, and the Heart to clear Heart Heat. Also, it enters and **benefits the GB to reduce jaundice.**

13. _____, like *Dan Shen*, it both invigorates and nourishes the Blood. It **relaxes the sinews and unblocks the channels** for Wind Damp *Bi* syndrome.

14. _____ invigorates Blood, regulates menses, and promotes lactation. (Additionally it is sometimes used for auricular acupuncture).

15. _____ regulates menses and promotes lactation, reduces swelling and promotes purulent discharge. Modern use is for **cancer and tumors, especially of the breast** (enters Liver & Stomach channels)

16. _____ is known for treating **Wind Damp Cold Bi in the upper extremities**, especially the **shoulder**. Modern research shows that it is a powerful anti-inflammatory.

17. _____ aggressively breaks up and drives out Blood stasis, and reduces immobile masses.

18. _____ invigorates Blood, reduces swelling and alleviates pain. Used to stop bleeding for excessive post-partum bleeding.

19. Heavy, dense & rich in minerals (like bones) & entering the Liver and Kidney channels, _____ **promotes the healing of bones and sinews** and is especially **helpful for healing fractures**.

Formulas

Warm Interior

Dang Gui Si Ni Tang Xiao Jian Zhong Tang Tong Mai Si Ni Tang Qi Gui
Zhi Wu Wu Tang Da Jian Zhong Tang Bai Tong Tang
Li Zhong Wan **Si Ni Tang** Shen Fu Tang
Wu Zhu Yu Tang Si Ni Jia Ren Shen Tang

Warm the Channels & Disperse Cold
1. Blood Bi syndrome with mild External Wind (characterized by relatively superficial numbness without pain):
(this above fx is *Gui Zhi Tang* + *Huang Qi, and – Zhi Gan Cao*)

2. Cold in the channels with underlying Blood Deficiency:
(Because there are no other indications of Yang deficiency, and the pulse is so thin it is almost imperceptible)

Warm the Middle & Disperse Cold
3. Middle Jiao (Yang) Deficient Cold:
Herb Ingredients (4):

4. Warms and tonifies the Liver & Stomach, descends rebellious Qi, stops vomiting.
Three presentations (all with primary Sx of Vomiting and Middle Jiao Deficient Cold)
     1. Cold from Stomach Deficiency (vomiting, pain, gnawing hunger)
     2. Cold from Stomach & Liver Deficiency (vertex HA, dry heaves, spitting clear fluids)
     3. Cold attacking the Middle Jiao affecting Kidney (diarrhea, cold hands & feet so
        unbearable he wants to die, HA, vomiting)
Fx:
Herb Ingredients (4):

5. Spasmodic abdominal pain due to internal injury (from overwork, poor eating habits etc):
Fx:
This fx is another formula:_____ + one herb _____

6. Middle Jiao Deficient Yang (root) with ascendant Yin Cold to the Interior (branch) manifesting as excruciating epigatsric and abdominal pain & severe vomiting:

Rescue Devastated Yang
7. Yang Deficiency with severe Yuan Qi Deficiency & sudden collapse of Yang Qi:

8. Kidney (& Spleen) Yang Deficiency with Internal Cold manifesting as cold extremities, vomiting, and diarrhea with undigested food:
Herb Ingredients (3):

Variations of the above formula (question 8)
9. Diarrhea ceases but extremities remain cold, add (1 herb):
Formula:

10. Unblocks Yang & Breaks up Yin accumulation (in lower part of body):

11. Shao Yin Cold with Exterior Heat manifesting same as principle formula with no aversion ot cold, and may have a flushed face, or the pulse may be imperceptible due to severe diarrhea:

WEEK 7

Meridian Symptom Review (Shanghai Text)

1. **High fever, tidal fevers, flushed face, sweating and delirium,** sometimes sensitivity to cold, or pain in the eyes, dry nostrils and nosebleed, fever blisters, sore throat, swelling on the neck, **facial paralysis** (mouth awry), chest pain, pain or distension along the course of the channel in the leg and foot, coldness in the lower limb:

2. Fever, parched mouth and thirst, sore throat, nosebleed, **toothache**, red and painful eyes, swelling of the neck, pain along the course of the channel on the upper arm, shoulder and shoulder blade, motor impairment of the fingers:

3. Stiff neck, spasms in the arm or leg, flushed face, pain in the eyes, subaxillary swelling, spasms and **contracture of the elbow and arm**, restricting movement, hot palms:

4. **Heaviness** in the body or head, general feverishness, fatigued limbs and **emaciated muscles**, stiffness of the tongue, coldness along the medial side of the leg and knee, edema in the foot or leg:

5. Pain along the lower vertebrae, low back pain, coldness in the feet, motor impairment or muscular atrophy of the foot, dryness in the mouth, sore throat, **pain in the sole of the foot** or along the posterior aspect of the lower leg or thigh:

6. Swelling an pain in the throat, pain in the cheek and jaw, **redness in the eyes, deafness**, pain behind the ear or along the lateral aspect of the shoulder and upper arm:

7. Headache, **vertigo, blurred vision, tinnitus,** fever, spasms in the extremities

8. Fever and sensitivity to cold, nasal congestion, headache, pain in the chest, clavicle, shoulder and back, chills and pain along the channel on the arm

9. General feverishness, headache, pain in the eyes, pain along the back of the upper arm, dry throat, thirst, hot or painful palms, coldness in the palms and soles of the feet, **pain along the scapula and/or medial aspect of the forearm:**

10. Numbness of the mouth and tongue, pain in the neck or cheek, sore throat, stiff neck, **pain along the lateral aspect of the shoulder** and upper arm.

11. (Alternating) **chills and fever, headache, stiff neck, pain in the lumbar region, nasal congestion, disease of the eye**, pain along the back of the leg and foot:

12.: Alternating fever and chills, headache, ashen complexion; pain in the eye or jaw, swelling in the sub-axillary region, scrofula, deafness, pain along the channel in the hip region, leg or foot:

1. Abdominal distension, fullness or edema, discomfort when reclining, seizures, persistent hunger, yellow urine.

2. Pain or fullness in chest and ribs or below ribs, irritability, shortness of breath, discomfort when reclining, vertigo, mental disorders

3. Coughing, asthma, shortness of breath, fullness in the chest, parched throat, changes in the color of urine, irritability, blood in the sputum, palms hot; sometimes accompanied by distended abdomen and loose stool.

4. Vertigo, facial edema, ashen complexion, blurred vision, shortness of breath, drowsiness and irritability, loose stool, chronic diarrhea or constipation, abdominal distension, vomiting, impotence.

5. Abdominal distension, hardness and fullness in the lower abdomen, enuresis, frequent urination, edema, dysuresis.

6. Abdominal pain, intestinal noises, loose stool; sometimes accompanied by shortness of breath and belching. (should include constipation)

7. Abdominal pain, fullness or distension, diarrhea, incomplete digestion of food, intestinal noises, vomiting, hard lumps in the abdomen, reduced appetite, jaundice, constipation.

8. Pain in the ribs, vomiting, bitter taste in the mouth, chest pain.

9. Pain and distension in the lower abdomen, possibly extending around the waist or to the genitals; diarrhea, or abdominal pain with 'dry' stool or constipation.

10. Pain in the lower abdomen, enuresis, retention of urine, painful urination, mental disorders.

11. Impaired speech, fainting, irritability, fullness in the chest, motor impairment of the tongue, palpitations, chest pain, mental disorders.

12. Fullness or pain in the costal region or chest, hard lumps in the upper abdomen, abdominal pain, vomiting, jaundice, loose stool, pain in the lower abdomen, hernia, enuresis, retention of urine, dark urine:

Meridians & Points
Meridians & Points
8 Extra Meridians
-facilitates the functional relationship among the Regular channels
-each has its own functional characteristics & sx

1. Sx: fullness in the abdomen, irregular menstruation, **leukorrhea**, pain in the lumbar region, weakness or motor impairment of the lower limb.
Channel:
Confluent Point:
3 Crossing Points:

2. Sx: diseases of the eyes, tightness and **spasms of the muscles along the lateral aspect of the lower leg** while those along the medial aspect are flaccid or atrophied (found in cases of **seizures** or paralysis), pain in the lumbar region, stiffness in the lumbar region
Channel:
Confluent Point:
Xi Cleft:

3. Sx: Liver & Kidney pathologies, problems with pregnancy, infertility, urogenital problems, leukorrhea, irregular menstruation, colic, etc
Channel:
Confluent Point:
Luo:

4. Sx: Chills and fever, vertigo; muscular fatigue, stiffness and pain, pain and distension in the waist
Channel:
Confluent Point:
Xi Cleft:

5. Sx: Because this channel arises in the pelvic cavity, it is intimately associated with gynecological disorders, and potentially male sexual irregularities including impotence as well.
Channel:
Confluent point:
Crossing Points:

6. Sx: chest, Heart, Stomach, Blood & Ying Qi related (none listed in Shanghai)
Channel:
Confluent Point:
Xi Cleft:

7. Sx: stiffness & pain along the **spinal column**, mental disorders, febrile disease, **Qi rushing upward** toward the Heart, colic, **constipation**, enuresis, hemorrhoids & infertility
Channel:
Confluent Point:
Crossing pts:

8. Sx: disease of the **eye, tightness and spasms of the muscles along the medial aspect of the lower leg** while those along the lateral aspect are flaccid or atrophied (found in cases of **seizures** or paralysis), lower abdominal pain, pain along the waist to the genitals, hernia, leukorrhagia
Channel:
Confluent Point:
Xi Cleft:

8 Extra Meridian Confluent Points

Indications:	Confluent Pt.	Channel (8 Extras)
Diseases of Heart, chest & Stomach		
Diseases of the inner canthus, neck, ear, shoulder S.I. & U.B.		
Dz of the outer canthus back of the ear, cheek, neck, & shoulder		
Disease of the respiratory system, chest & diaphragm		

Intimate relationship with Kidney Yang:
Connects with Yin Meridians:
Ensures pregnancy:
Closely related to pre-natal & post-natal Qi:
Sea of Yin & Yang Qi (2 channels):
Connects with Yang Meridians:
3 Extra Meridians affect the Kidney, connect to the pelvic area & uterus, and are especially
        important for female reproduction and male sexual function:
Not directly connected to the uterus but affects the holding function:
Surrounding back pain (back to hypochondrium to abdomen):
Used for internal organ pain, nausea, vomiting, abdominal pain:
Dominates Wei Qi (reaches skin, hair, muscles and tendons):
Good for common cold:
Leukorrhea, prolapse, heavy bleeding:
Connects with the eyes (3 channels):
Always excited, cannot sleep (eyes open), madness:
Sea of 12 regular meridians (& Sea of Blood):
Dominates medial & lateral sides (esp of legs):
3 meridians that connect to the pelvis:
Connects to the brain (3 channels):
Depressed & sleepy:
Lump in abdomen:
3 channels for dry itchy throat (connect with the throat):
Hernia: (+ which 2 regular channels for hernia:)
2 channels for hemorrhoid:
Closely associated with Ying Qi:

Front *Mu*

Lu ___   Sp ___   Ht ___   Kid ___   P ___   Liv ___
LI ___   St ___   SI ___   UB ___   SJ ___   GB ___

1. Abdominal distension, borborygmus, pain in the hypochondriac region, vomiting, diarrhea, indigestion:

2. Enuresis, nocturnal emission, frequency of urination, retention of urine, hernia, irregular menstruation, morbid leukorrhea, dysmenorrhea, uterine bleeding, postpartum hemorrhage, lower abdominal pain, indigestion, diarrhea, prolapse of the rectum, flaccid type of apoplexy:

3. Enuresis, nocturnal emission, impotence, hernia, uterine bleeding, irregular menstruation, dysmenorrhea, morbid leukorrhea, frequency of urination, retention of urine, pain in the lower abdomen, prolapse of the uterus, vaginitis:

4. Abdominal distension, borborygmus, diarrhea, pain in the lumbar and hypochondriac region:

5. Pain in the hypochondriac region, vomiting, acid regurgitation, hiccup, jaundice, mastitis:

6. Hypochondriac pain, abdominal distension, hiccup, acid regurgitaiton, mastitis, depression, febrile diseases:

7. Abdominal pain, diarrhea, edema, hernia, anuria, enuresis, amenorrhea, morbid leukorrhea, uterine bleeding, postpartum hemorrhage:

8. Asthma, pain in the chest, fullness in the chest, palpitation, **insufficient lactation**, hiccup, difficulty in swallowing:

9. Pain in the cardiac region and the chest, nausea, acid regurgitation, difficulty in swallowing, vomiting, mental disorders, epilepsy, palpitation:

10. Abdominal pain and distension, borborygmus, pain around the umbilicus, constipation, diarrhea, dysentery, irregular menstruation, edema:

11. Stomachache, abdominal distension, borborygmus, nausea, vomiting, acid regurgitation, diarrhea, dysentery, jaundice, indigestion, insomnia:

12. Cough, asthma, pain in the chest, shoulder and arm, fullness in the chest:

Back *Shu*

Lu ___   Sp ___   Ht ___   Kid ___   P ___   Liv ___
LI ___   St ___   SI ___   UB ___   SJ ___   GB ___

1. Jaundice, bitter taste of the mouth, pain in the chest and hypchondriac region, **pulmonary tuberculosis**, afternoon fever:

2. Jaundice, pain in the hypochondriac region, redness of the eye, blurring of vision, night blindness, mental disorders, epilepsy, backache, spitting of blood, epistaxis:

3. Epigastric pain, abdominal distension, jaundice, vomiting, diarrhea, dysentery, bloody stools, profuse menstruation, edema, anorexia, backache:

4. Cough, asthma, chest pain, spitting of blood, afternoon fever, night sweating:

5. Pain in the chest and hypochondriac and epigastric regions, anorexia, abdominal distension, borborygmus, diarrhea, nausea, vomiting:

6. Cardiac pain, panic, loss of memory, palpitation, cough, spitting of blood, nocturnal emission, **night sweating,** mania, epilepsy:

7. Cough, cardiac pain, palpitation, stuffy chest, vomiting:

8. Borborygmus, abdominal distension, indigestion, vomiting, diarrhea, dysentery, edema, pain and stiffness of the lower back:

9. Nocturnal emission, impotence, enuresis, irregular menstruation, leukorrhea, low back pain, weakness of the knee, blurring of vision, dizziness, tinnitus, deafness, edema, asthma, diarrhea:

10. **Retention of urine, enuresis, frequent urination**, diarrhea, constipation, stiffness and pain of the lower back:

11. Low back pain, borborygmus, abdominal distension, diarrhea, constipation, muscular atrophy, pain, numbness and motor impairment of the lower extremities, sciatica:

12. Lower abdominal pain and distension, dysentery, nocturnal emission, hematuria, enuresis, morbid leukorrhea, lower back pain, sciatica:

Tai Yang- general sx:
P:

Tai Yang Cold (Exterior Excess Cold)
Distinguishing Sx:
P:
Other Sx:
Fx:

Tai Yang Wind Invading (Exterior Deficient Cold Syndrome)
Distinguishing Sx:
P:
Other Sx:
Fx:

Yang Ming (Excess Heat Syndrome)

Yang Ming Channel Syndrome
Organs involved:
Sx:
T:
P:
Fx:

Yang Ming Organ Syndrome
Organs involved:
Sx:

T:
P:
Fx:

Shao Yang (half interior, half exterior syndrome)
Organs/channels:
Zheng Qi is weak, Pathogen is strong
Sx:

T:
P:
Fx:

Tai Yin Syndrome (Deficient Cold Syndrome)
Organs:
Sx:

T:
P:
Fx:

Shao Yin
Organs/channels:

<u>Shao Yin Cold Syndrome</u>
Main Sx:

P:
T:
Other Sx:
If severe: coma or Yang collapse & P: minute (*wei mai*), no root
Fx:

<u>Shao Yin Heat Syndrome</u>
Sx:
T:
P:
Fx:

Jue Yin
Organs/channels:
Complicated involving Heat, Cold, Excess & Deficiency
Sx:
Fx:
(If vomiting roundworms then Fx:)

<u>6 External Evils</u>

1.   3.   5.
2.   4.   6.

The primary External factor in causing disease:
Abdominal distension, fullness,, poor appetite:
Yang pathogen characterized by upward movement:
Impairs opening and closing of pores:
Often consumes Yin causing thirst with desire to drink:
HA, nasal obstruction, itching or pain in the throat, sweating, facial edema:
Yang pathogen characterized by extreme Heat, "4 Bigs":
Yin factor causing contraction and stagnation:
Yin pathogen impairs Yang and easily obstructs Qi circulation:
Dry nose and throat, dry mouth with thirst, chapped skin:
Migratory symptoms, abrupt onset, itching:
Weeping eczema, suppurating sores, profuse purulent leukorrhea, turbid urine:
Spasmodic contraction of tendons, impaired circulation of qi and blood:
Yang factor easily invades upper part of body, head and face:
Predominant Qi of Summer, only seen in own season:
Sunstroke, sudden collapse and coma:
Deviation of mouth and eyes, facial spasms:
Pain, lack of sweating, restricted movement:
Fixed Bi:
Migrating Bi:
Constipation and reduced urination:
Impaired Lung function, causing dry cough with scanty sticky or bloody sputum:
Tongue ulcers, swollen painful gums, restlessness, mania, coma:
Dizziness, vertigo, tetanus:
Heaviness & turbidity:
Carbuncles, furuncles, boils and ulcers:

week 7

Herbs
(Warm Herbs)
Transform Cold Phlegm

Ban Xia	*Bai Qian*
Tian Nan Xing (& Dan Nan Xing)	*Bai Jie Zi*
Bai Fu Zi	*Jie Geng*
Xuan Fu Hua	*Zao Jiao*

1. From Southern China _____ lives in cool moist habitat, precisely what it is good at transforming. It is warm, pungent, and poisonous until it is processed, enters the Spleen and Stomach to **dry Damp and transform Phlegm in the Middle Jiao**. The true version of this herb, *Pinellia Ternata* **descends Stomach Qi** for nausea and vomiting, and is used for copious white sputum. (It is one of the two "aged" herbs in "Two Aged Decoction", *Er Chen Tang*)

2. Neutral in nature, _____ can be used for either hot or cold conditions. It expels phlegm, stops cough, and benefits the throat. It is added to prescriptions to treat edema because it opens and disperses Lung Qi, described as opening the lid of the tea pot to facilitate the surge of water flow." Also **guides to the Lung.**

3. _____ descends both Lung Qi and expels phlegm and descends Stomach Qi to stop vomiting. It is the one of the few flowers that descends.

4. _____ is acrid, sweet, and slightly warm. It expels phlegm and descends rebellious Qi, for copious sputum, regardless of Cold or Heat patterns. It is often combined with *Qian Hu* for **cough**.

5. _____ has a strong effect to expel Wind Phlegm from the Head for facial paralysis post stroke. Also, it can be applied topically to relieve toxicity and dissipate nodules. It is contraindicated in pregnancy.

6. _____ Is similar to *Ban Xia* but much more drying. It mainly enters the Liver channel to treat Wind Phlegm. Raw it is used for topical application only, and is contraindicated in pregnancy.

7. Bitter and cool, _____ is primarily used for Phlegm Heat with cough, and **Phlegm Heat causing contractions, seizures, convulsions, and mania.**

8. Acrid and warm, _____ is used to treat Lung Phlegm Cold with Qi accumulation, Phlegm Cold channel obstruction, and Phlegm Cold nodules and swellings.

9. Acrid, warm and slightly toxic, _____ strongly dispels phlegm, opens orifices to revive the *shen*, dissipates clumps and reduces swellings. Additionally, Bensky suggests using it as a suppository to unblock the bowel and expel roundworms.

Transform Phlegm Heat

Qian Hu	Gua Lou Ren	Hai Ge Ke
Chuan Bei Mu	(Tian Hua Fen)	Kun Bu
Zhe Bei Mu	Tian Zhu Huang	Hai Zao
Quan Gua Lou	Zhu Li	Pang Da Hai
(aka Gua Lou Shi)	Zhu Ru	Huang Yao Zi
Gua Lou Pi	Fu Hai Shi	

These two herbs are bitter and cold, enter the Lung and Heart channels. They both can **transform phlegm Heat, dissipate nodules and treat cough with thick, green sputum that is difficult to expectorate**, with dryness in the mouth.

1. _____ is sweet and is less cold. Sweet and cold generate Yin, and so it **moistens the Lung, for Phlegm Heat with Lung Yin Deficiency**.

2. _____ is more bitter and colder, and has no function of moistening. It is **stronger in clearing Heat, reducing Fire, and breaking up congealed Phlegm**. (Combined with other herbs it is used to treat tumors).

The following **three herbs come from bamboo**. They are sweet and cold, and have the functions of clearing Heat and transforming Phlegm.

3. _____ enters the Heart and Liver, and is **effective for dislodging phlegm, clearing Heat, cooling the Heart and controlling convulsions**.

4. _____ is the coldest, enters the Heart. Lung and Stomach, has a **lubricating** nature and **strongly eliminates Phlegm Heat, especially when it blocks the meridians** (as in epilepsy, facial paralysis, and numbness of the limbs). It also **opens the Heart orifice** (for Phlegm Heat disturbing the mind).

5. _____ is slightly cold, enters the Lung, Stomach and Gall Bladder meridians, and besides clearing Heat and transforming Phlegm, it is effective for **dispersing constrained Qi, eliminating irritability and calming the Mind.** It soothes the Stomach Qi and clears Heat for nausea and vomiting.

The following four herbs come from the plant *Tricosanthes*.
The first two are sweet, bitter, and cold. They enter the lung, Stomach and LI, clear Heat from the Lung, transform Phlegm Heat and unbind Chest Qi. The also promote bowel movement and treat constipation. Of these two,

6. _____ is **stronger at clearing Heat and transforming phlegm.**

7. _____ is **stronger in moistening the intestine and promoting bowel movement**.
A third part of the plant, _____ is sweet and cold (like *Chuan Bei Mu*) and therefore has a **moistening function of the Lung and throat** (for hoarseness, sore throat, and thirst due to Lung Dryness). It is not as strong as the above two herbs at clearing Heat.

8. The last part of this plant that we use as a medicinal herb, _____ is in a different category. It is bitter, sour, cold and slightly sweet, has no function of transforming Phlegm but it can **clear Heat from the Lung, generate Body Fluids, and alleviate thirst**. It is contraindicated in pregnancy (note: *Luo Han Guo* is safe to relieve thirst for pregnant women)

The following two herbs are salty and cold (like their ocean home), and enter the Liver, Lung and Kidney. They transform Phlegm Heat, **soften hardness, dissipate nodules**, promote urination and reduce edema. They are often used together to treat scrofula and goiter.

9. _____ is stronger in transforming Phlegm and dissipating nodules (for goiter and scrofula)

10. _____ is stronger in softening hardness and reducing congealed blood (for hepatosplenomegaly, Liver cirrhosis, and tumors)

11. _____ is bitter, acrid and slightly cold. It is **more often used for Wind Heat patterns, though it can be used for Wind Cold as well** (especially combined with *Bai Qian*)

12. Bitter, salty, and neutral, _____ clears Phlegm Heat, descends Lung Qi, softens hardness and dissipates nodules, promotes urination and expels Dampness (turbid urinary dysfunction). Additionally in its calcined (*duan*) form it is used **for acid regurgitation.**

13. Similar to the above herb (question 12), _____ clears Phlegm Heat from the Lungs, softens hardness, dissipates nodules. However, it is salty and cold (not neutral) and so it promotes urination for **hot or stony painful urinary dysfunction**.

14. To clear and disseminate Lung Qi **for sore throat, infuse** _____. Also clears the Intestines to unblock the bowel. To encourage the expression of rashes, apply topically.

15. Bitter and neutral, _____ dissipates nodules, reduces masses, cools the Blood and stops bleeding, and can be applied topically to reduce toxic swellings.

Stop Wheezing

Xing Ren	*Bai Bu*
Zi Wan	*Sang Bai Pi*
Kuan Dong Hua	*Ting Li Zi*
Su Zi	*Ma Dou Ling*
Pi Pa Ye	*Mu Hu Die*

1. _____ is indicated for **cough & wheezing regardless of pathology** (external or internal, heat or cold, deficiency or excess). The more frequently used norther variety (*bei*) is a bitter (*ku*) more strongly descends the Qi to effectively stop cough and calm wheezing. It is slightly toxic.
*The southern variety (*Nan*) also called Sweet (*Tian*) is more nourishing and mostiening, more for deficiency and more common in cooking recipes.

Sang Bai Pi & Ting Li Zi both drain pathogens for the Lungs and calm wheezing. They promote urination and reduce swelling.
2. _____ is less potent in promoting urination, used for mild edema and t drains heat from the Lung
3. _____ strongly promotes urination for severe edema, and drains stagnation and blockage of Lung Qi.

Zi Wan, Bai Bu, & Kuang Dong Hua all exclusively enter the Lung channel, moisten the Lung and descent Qi, transform phlegm and stop coughing. They are commonly combined to treat all patterns of cough, especially effective for chornic deficient type.
4. _____ has an additional function of expelling parasites and killing lice.
5. _____ is relatively stronger at stopping cough.
6. _____ strongly transforms phlegm (raw for esternal conditions, honey fried for Lung deficiency with chronic cough)

7. Bitter and cool, _____ enters the Lung to calm coughing and resolve phlegm, and enters the Stomach to clear Heat and descend rebellious Qi (honey-fried for cough and raw for vomiting)

8. _____ enters the Lung to descend Lung Qi and resolve phlegm & Qi stagnation with coughing and wheezing. It also enters the Large Intestine channel to moisten the Intestines.

Formulas: *Tonifying*

Si Jun Zi Tang   *Zhi Gan Cao Tang*   *Zuo Gui Wan*
Shen Ling Bai Zhu San   *Ba Zhen Tang*   *Shi Hu Ye Guang Wan*
Bu Zhong Yi Qi Tang   **Shi Quan Da Bu Tang**   **Jin Gui Shen Qi Wan**
Sheng Mai San   **Liu Wei Di Huang Wan**   *You Gui Wan*
Si Wu Tang   *(Qi Jui Di Huang Wan)*
Shao Yo Gan Cao Tang   *(Zhi Bai Di Huang Wan)*
Gui Pi Tang   *(Mai Wei Di Huang Wan)*

Tonify Qi:
1. Spleen Qi Deficiency leading to internally generated Dampness:

2. Deficiency of Spleen & Stomach Qi leading to sinking of the Yang:

3. Classic presentation of deficient Spleen Qi, usually caused by improper eating, excessive deliberation or overwork:

4. Concurrent deficiency of Qi & Yin, primarily of the Lungs:

Tonify Blood
5. Originally used for when inappropriate use of sweating had injured the Liver Blood or Yin. Today used for any type of pain (esp in the calves) with blood deficiency or injury to the Fluids:

6. Blood deficiency, primarily of the Liver:

Tonify Qi & Blood
7. Primary inury to the Spleen, and therefore the Blood becomes deficient and unable to nourish the Heart. (The Spleen stores the *yi* and the Heart the *shen*, and so inability to concentrate is one of the main sx):

8. Another consumptive condition of Qi & Blood. The Heart is undernourished, therefore giving the *shen* no place to reside. Irregular pulse is one of the key Sx:

9. Another consumptive condition of Qi & Blood, most often due to chronic disease or excessive Blood loss:

The above formula is two formulas combined: _____ & _____

10. For Qi & Blood deficiency with a predominance of deficient Qi tending toward Cold:

The above formula is Ba Zhen Tang + (two herbs) _____ & _____

Nourish & Tonify Yin
11. Classic presentation of Kidney & Liver Yin Deficiency:

12. Visual disorders due to Liver/Kidney Yin Deficiency leading to deficient Fire and Wind:

13. Kidney Deficiency of both Yin & Essence

Warm & Tonify Yang
14. Classic presentation of Kidney Yang Deficiency (with deficient Ming Men Fire)
*this formula warms and tonifies Kidney Yang

15. Kidney Yang Deficiency (with Jing Def):
*this formula warms and tonifies Kidney Yang, replenishes *jing* essence & tonifies Blood

Channel	6 Stages	Begins:	Organ Connections: (all connect to self and paired organ)	Other Connections
Lung	Hand Tai Yin			
Large Intestine				
Stomach				
Spleen				
Heart				
Small Intestine				
Urinary Bladder				
Kidney				
Pericardium				
San Jiao				
Gallbladder				
Liver				
Du	n/a			
Ren	n/a			
Chong	n/a			
Dai	n/a			
Yang Qiao	n/a			
Yin Qiao	n/a			
Yang Wei	n/a			
Yin Wei	n/a			

Extra Points

1. Located at the lateral ¼ and the medial ¾ of the infraorbital margin:

2. Indicated for hepatosplenomegaly & lumbar pain, *Pi Gen* is located ____ cun lateral to ____.

3. *An Mian*, location & indication: midway between:

4. *Ding Chuan* is _____ cun lateral to (point)_____ , at the level of _____

5. *Zi Gong Xue* is ____ cun lateral to (point)____ , _____ cun above the pubic symphysis

6. *Luo Zhen* indication:

7. *Yao Tong Xue* (for acute lumbar sprain), location:

8. *Yao Yan* is ____ to ____ cun lateral to ____ , parallel with which back *shu* point ____

9. *Jian Qian*, for shoulder pain & upper extremities paralysis, is located midway between _____ and
_____

10. Main extra point for hemorrhoids:_____
& location: _____ cun above _____on either side of _____

11. For appendicitis, what extra point might you use?
    Location: tender spot about ____ cun below _____

12. For inflammation of the gallbladder (acute or chronic), gallstones, or worms in the bile duct, what point might you use?
    Location: tender spot ____ cun below _____

13. The "knee eyes", or in Chinese _____ are located medial and lateral to the _____

14. Which extra points are located on the web between the toes: And on the web between the fingers (clears heat):

15. For malnutrition, bleed which points?
16. *Bi Tong* is located: at the highest point of the nasolabial groove
    and is often needled from _____

17. *Hua Tuo Jia Ji* points are located ____ cun from the midline, and they range from which vertebrae to which vertebrae?

18. Located at the depression of the midpoint of the superior patellar border:
19. Indicated for rubella, eczema, and castrointestinal parasitic diseases, which extra point?
    Location: ____ cun above _____

(Meridian Theory as per Shanghai Text)

Luo Channels
How many channels?
Major function:
Do they have independent points along the channel?

Divergent Channels
Function:
Do they have independent points along the channel?
Independent Sx?

Minute Connecting
Connect to tissue
(many)

Blood Superficial
Just under skin
(many)

Cutaneous Regions
Follow Regular Meridians
Most superficial, on skin
Internal organ problem can reflect skin sensitivity

Muscle-Tendon Channels
How many?
Relate to:
Do they have independent points along the channel?

Muscle Meridian Meeting Points
3 arm yang:
3 leg yang:
3 arm yin:
3 leg yin:

Zang Fu Syndrome Differentiaton (CAM '87: p. 288-310)

Heart Blood Defiency   Heart Yin Deficiency

compare

contrast

Heart Fire   Heart Yin Def

compare

contrast

Heart Phlegm   Heart Phlegm Heat

compare

contrast

Lung Wind Cold   Lugn Qi Deficiency

compare

contrast

Spleen Qi Deficiency   Spleen Yang Deficiency

compare

contrast

Liver Yang Rising   Liver Fire

compare

contrast

week 8

Auricular Acupuncture
(Shanghai 472-491, CAM 531-550)

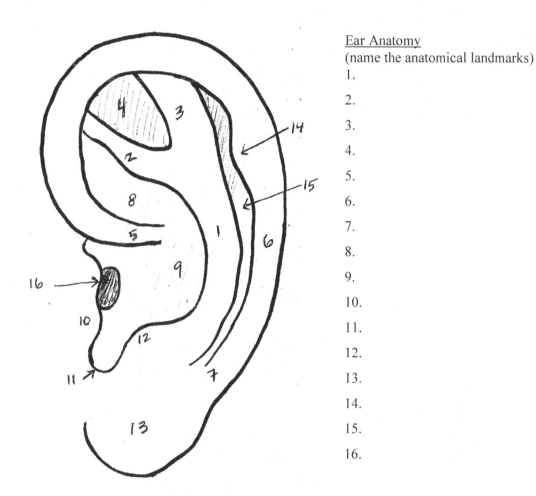

Ear Anatomy
(name the anatomical landmarks)
1.
2.
3.
4.
5.
6.
7.
8.
9.
10.
11.
12.
13.
14.
15.
16.

Be able to locate the following important acupuncture points:

Helix: diaphragm, anus, ext genitalia, hemrrhoid (p. 479)
Scapha: fingers, wrist, allergy, shoulder, elbow, shoulder joint (p. 480)
Crus of antehelix: toes, ankle, heel, knee, kneejoint, hoip joint,
　　sympathetic (p. 481)
Antehelix: sciatic nerve, lumbar vertebrae, abdomen, lumbago, neck, sacrum,
　　thoracic vertebrae, cervical vertebrae (p. 482)
Tragus & Antigragus: heart, adrenal, thirst, hunger, hupertension, throat,
　　inner nose, forehead(p. 482)
Antitragus & Intertragic notch: occiput, temple, vertex, stop wheezing, brain,
　　brain stem, endocrine (p. 484)
Antitragus: ovaries, subcoretex, hormone, testicles, pituitary (p. 485)
Triangular Fossa: uterus, neurogate (aka *shenmen*), wheezing, hip joint (p. 485-6)
Cavum & Cymba Conchae: mouth, esophagus, stomach, duodenum,
　　small intestine, large instestine, prostate, bladder, kidney (p. 486-7)
Cavum & Cymba Conchae: pancreas, liver, gallbladder, spleen, heart (p. 488)
Cavum & Cymba Conchae: upper lung, lower lung, bronchi, trachea (p. 489)

Homunculus
(image of a human body
super-imposed over the ear)

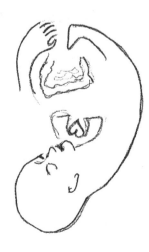

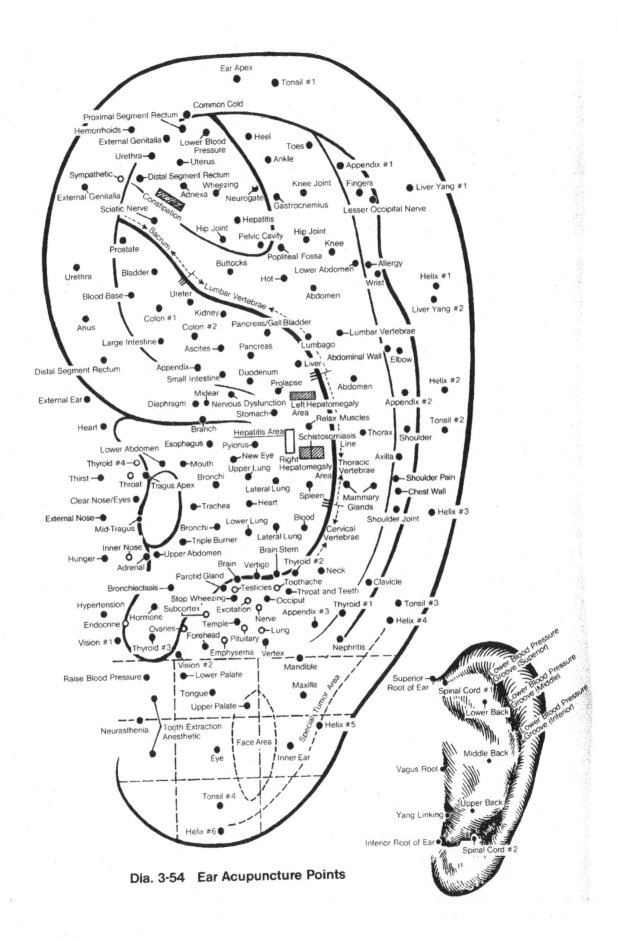

Dia. 3-54 **Ear Acupuncture Points**

Scalp (Shanghai 497-501)

1. The midline of the head is measured from the _____ to the _____
2. 0.5 cm behind the midline is the _____
3. For the motor and sensory area lines, the upper 1/5 is related to the _____
4. And the second and third 2/5's are related to the _____
5. And the lower two fifths are related to the _____
6. With the tuber parietale origin, three needles can be inserted inferiorly, anteriorly and posteriorly to a length of 3 cm. This are is _____

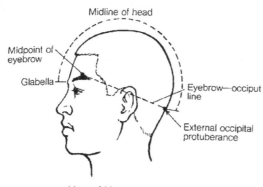

Midline of head
Midpoint of eyebrow
Glabella
Eyebrow—occiput line
External occipital protuberance

Lines of Measurement

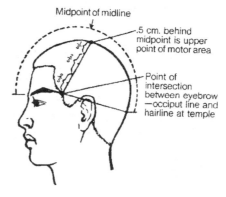

Midpoint of midline
.5 cm. behind midpoint is upper point of motor area
Point of intersection between eyebrow —occiput line and hairline at temple

Motor Area Measurements

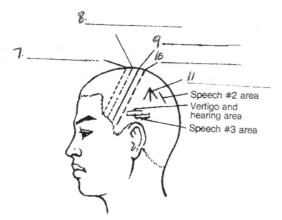

8. _____
9. _____
7. _____
10. _____
11. _____
Speech #2 area
Vertigo and hearing area
Speech #3 area

Stimulation Areas—Side View

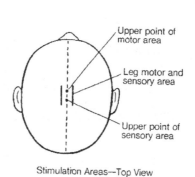

Upper point of motor area
Leg motor and sensory area
Upper point of sensory area

Stimulation Areas—Top View

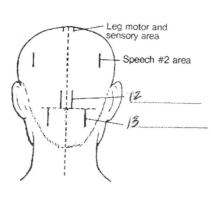

Leg motor and sensory area
Speech #2 area
12. _____
13. _____

Stimulation Areas—Back View

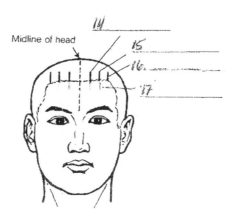

Midline of head
14. _____
15. _____
16. _____
17. _____

Stimulation Areas—Front View

Calm Shen

herb (yao 藥)	flavor (wei 味)		temp (qi 氣)	channels					
Anchor & Calm Shen									
Long Gu	**sweet**	astringent	**neutral**	**Ht**	**K**	Liv			
(Mu Li)	salty	astringent	**cool**		**K**	Liv			
Ci Shi	acrid, salty		**cold**		**K**	Liv			
Zhu Sha	sweet	toxic	**cool**	**Ht**					
(Zhen Zhu)	sweet, salty		**cold**	**Ht**		Liv			
Hu Po	sweet		**neutral**	**Ht**		Liv		UB	

Nourish & Calm Shen									
suan zao ren	sweet, sour		**neutral**	**Ht**		Liv	Sp	GB	
bai zi ren	sweet		**neutral**	**Ht**	K		Sp	LI	
yuan zhi	bitter, acrid		**sl. warm**	Ht					Lu
he huan pi	sweet		neutral	Ht		Liv			
ye jiao teng	sweet, sl. bitter		neutral	Ht		Liv			

OPEN ORIFICES

herb (yao 藥)	flavor (wei 味)		temp (qi 氣)	channels					
she xiang	**acrid**	**aromatic**	warm	**Ht**	**Sp**	Liv			
su he xiang	**acrid,** sweet	**aromatic**	warm	**Ht**	**Sp**				
bing pian	**acrid,** bitter		cool	**Ht**	**Sp**		Lu		
shi chang pu	**acrid**	**aromatic**	sl. warm	**Ht**			St		

EXTINGUISH WIND

herb (yao 藥)	flavor (wei 味)		temp (qi 氣)	channels					
ling yang jiao	salty		cold	Ht	**Liv**				
gou teng	sweet		cool	Ht	**Liv**				
tian ma	sweet		neutral		**Liv**				
bai ji li	acrid, bitter		warm		**Liv**	Lu			
shi jue ming	salty		cold		**Liv**	K			
di long	salty		cold		**Liv**	Lu		UB	Sp
quan xie	salty, acrid	toxic	neutral		**Liv**				
wu gong	acrid	toxic	warm		**Liv**				
jiang can	acrid, salty		neutral		**Liv**	Lu			
mu li	salty	astringent	cool		**Liv**	K	(anchor, calm spirit)		
dai zhe shi	bitter		cold	**Ht**	**Liv**	(anchor, calm spirit)			Pc

TONIFY QI

herb (yao 藥)	flavor (*wei* 味)		temp (qi 氣)	channels							
ren shen	**sweet,** sl. bitter		sl. warm	**Lu**	**Sp**						
dang shen	**sweet**		neutral	**Lu**	**Sp**						
tai zi shen	**sweet,** sl. bitter		neutral	**Lu**	**Sp**						
huang qi	**sweet**		sl. warm	**Lu**	**Sp**						
shan yao	**sweet**		neutral	**Lu**	**Sp**	K					
bai zhu	bitter, **sweet**		warm		**Sp**		St				
da zao	**sweet**		neutral		**Sp**		St				
gan cao, sheng	**sweet**		neutral	**Lu**	**Sp**		St	Ht	(all 12)		
gan cao, zhi	**sweet**		warm	**Lu**	**Sp**		St	Ht	(all 12)		
huang jing	**sweet**		neutral	**Lu**	**Sp**	K					
yi tang	**sweet**		sl. warm	**Lu**	**Sp**		St				
bai bian dou	**sweet**		neutral		**Sp**		St		(clear summer heat)		
xi yang shen	**sweet,** sl. bitter		cold	**Lu**		K		Ht	(tonify yin)		

Herbs: *Calm Spirit*

Anchor & Calm Spirit		**_Nourish & Calm Spirit_**	
Long Gu	*Zhu Sha*	**Suan Zao Ren**	*He Huan Pi*
(Mu Li)	*(Zhen Zhu)*	*Bai Zi Ren*	*Ye Jiao Teng*
Ci Shi	*Hu Po*	*Yuan Zhi*	

The following two herbs both **pacify the Liver and calm the Mind.** They also **both astringe and can stabilize the Essence and Body Fluids.**

1. _____ is **stronger at sedating the Heart Spirit** and calming the Mind. It is sweet and neutral.

2. _____ is salty and cold, and is stronger at reducing Heat in order to calm the Mind. It has an additional function of **softening hardness** and dissipating Phlegm.

The five nourishing herbs in this category are particularly good **calming the Spirit** for **chronic insomnia.**

3. _____ is sweet and Sour, enters primarily the Liver. Sweetness can to**nify the Liver & Heart Blood** and sour can **stabilize Qi & Blood.** (For "calm spirit" function, *chao* form is best)

4. _____ primarily enters the Heart channel. It is sweet and **moistening**, nourishes Heart Blood, and stops sweating.

5. _____ is sweet & neutral, **tonifies Blood**, calms the Spirit and **opens the channels.** It is especially good for conditions of the Blood being too weak to circulate properly. (It is the vine of *Polygonum Multiflorum*, where _____ is the tuber/root)

6. _____ is sweet & neutral, enters Heart, Spleen and Lung channels. It regulates Chest Qi & calms Spirit, especially suitable for patients who suffer from **depression** as well as insomnia.

7. _____ is pungent to disperse, and bitter to descend. It is good at removing **Phlegm** and improving the Heart-Kidney connection. (Careful with dosage, as too much can irritate the gastric mucosa, cause nausea and increase respiratory tract secretions)

Zhu Sha, Hu Po, & *Zhen Zhu* are all used in treating palpitations and emotional distress.

8. _____ has the ability to **invigorate the blood** and dissipate stasis.

9. _____ is used **for seizures and convulsions** from high fever.

10. _____ is preferred in cases resulting from fright and anxiety.

11. _____ anchors and calms the Spirit, nourishes the Kidneys and augments the Liver, and aids the Kidneys in grasping the Qi.

Open Orifices

She Xiang   *Bing Pian*
Su He Xiang   *Shi Chang Pu*

She Xiang & Su He Xiang are used to open the orifices and treat loss of consciousness.
1. _____ is the **most intensely aromatic** and penetrating substance in the material medica.
2. _____ is especially useful for Wind Stroke with collapse due to phlegm.

3. _____ , one of Dr. Fu's preferred herbs, **opens the orifices, vaporizes phlegm and quiets the spirit.** It transforms turbid Dampness and harmonizes the Middle Jiao, and is used for Wind Cold Damp Bi (internally & topically)

4. _____ is acrid, bitter and cool, and is used for fainting and convulsions. It is applied topically for pain and swelling of the throat, and for sores and scabies.

Extinguish Wind

Ling Yang Jiao   *Quan Xie*
Gou Teng   *Wu Gong*
Tian Ma   *Jiang Can*
Bai Ji Li   *Mu Li (Anchor, calm Spirit)*
Shi Jue Ming   *Dai Zhe Shi (Anchor, calm Spirit)*
Di Long

Gou Teng and Tian Ma have similar properties of treating HA, dizziness, and vertigo, and are often used in combination.
1. _____ is sweet, warm, and dry, and is more often used in Wind Cold accompanied by Phlegm Damp.
2. _____ is sweet and cold, and is more often used in treating Heat induced Wind.

3. _____ enters the Blood level and strongly relieves toxicity. It can also be used in treating various manifestations of **Blood Heat.**

Quan Xie, Wu Gong and *Di Long* all extinguish Liver Wind, reliev spasms and control tremor.
4. _____ is salty and cold. It is milder at extinguishing Wind, but it clears Liver Heat the strongest. It particularly enters the collaterals (for Bi syndrome) and has been shown to stop wheezing.
5. _____ & _____ are **pungent and toxic,** and are almost identical in their **strong function of extinguishing Liver Wind**, relieving spasms and stopping pain.

6. Another insect, _____ extinguishes Wind, transforms Phlegm, and stops itching.

7. _____ dispels wind to **stop itching, brightens the Eyes,** and anchors Liver Yang.

8. _____ strongly descends rebellious Qi, anchors floating Liver Yang, clears Liver Fire, and Cools the Blood to stop bleeding.

9. _____ settles and calms the Spirit & **softens hardness.**

10. _____ drains Fire, **descends Yang and improves vision** (as do other herbs with this character in its name)

Tonify Qi

Ren Shen   Shan Yao   Huang Jing
Dang Shen   Bai Zhu   Yi Tang
Tai Zi Shen   Da Zao   Bai Bian Dou *(clear summer heat)*
Huang Qi   Gan Cao   Xi Yang Shen *(nourish yin)*

1. _____ **strengthens the Spleen**, for chronic diarrhea. It is sweet and neutral, but clears **summer heat.**

These two herbs were recognized as one entity in ancient times (until the *Ben Cao Cong Xin*, 1757 C.E.).
2. _____ is used for chronic and mild Qi deficiency.
3. _____ is used for **severe collapsed Qi and devastated Yang**.

4. _____ strengthens the Spleen and tonifies the Lung. Characterized by raising the Yang Qi, it is the **imperial herb for treating sunken Spleen Qi.** Additionally it consolidates the surface and **augments the Wei Qi** to stop spontaneous sweating (with *Bai Zhu & Fang Feng*). Finally, it promotes urination and generates tissue.

5. _____ is sweet and warm to **tonify the Middle Jiao Qi**, and bitter to **dry Damp**. Use raw to dry Dampness (for arthritis) and *chao* to tonify Spleen Qi.

6. _____ is sweet and cold. It **tonifies the Qi and nourishes the Yin**. Simmer separately for a long time before adding into the strained decoction.

7. _____ tonifies the Qi and Yin of the Lung, Spleen and Kidney. It is **stabilizing and binding**, and used to treat leakage (therefore use with caution with patients that tend towards constipation).

8. Due to its broad usage of **harmonizing** and integrating the actions of other herbs, _____ is said to **enter all 12 channels**. It is sweet to strengthen the Spleen and Mositen the Lung. It relieves pain & spasms (with *Bai Shao*). **Raw to clear toxicity**, *zhi* (honey-fried) for all other purposes.

9. Commonly combined with *Sheng Jiang* for mutual assistance, _____ can moderate the pungent and moving nauture of *Sheng Jiang,* while *Sheng Jiang* can balance lout the accumulative effects of this herb. Together they harmonize the *Ying & Wei.*

10. In traditional textbooks _____ is categorized into Yin Tonics. It tonifies Spleen Qi, augments Stomach Yin, and Yin of the Lung, Spleen and Kidney, and moistens the Lung.

11. Sweet, warm and moist _____ tonifies Qi and moderates spasm. Dissolve it into the strained decoction.

12. _____ mildly tonifies Spleen & Lung Qi, and nourishes the Yin to generate fluid.

Gua Lou & Xie Bai
One moistens and loosens
The other dissipates and frees the flow
Together they effectively
free the flow of Yang and move Qi,
Loosen the chest and clear the Lungs,
Transform Phlegm and scatter nodulation,
Stop pain and moisten the intestines to unblock the bowl
> *Gua Lou Xie Bai Bai Jiu Tang*
> *Gua Lou Xie Bai Ban Xia Tang*
> *Zhi Shi Gua Lou Gui Zhi Tang*

Zhi Shi & Hou Po **(from week 3)**
Zhi Shi dissipates clumps and reduces focal distension.
Hou Po disseminates Qi and relieves the sensation of fullness.
Together they **promote bowel movement by moving Qi.**
> *Da Cheng Qi Tang,*
> *Xiao Cheng Qi Tang,*
> *Ma Zi Ren Wan*
> *Zhi Shi Gua Lou Gui Zhi Tang*

Gao Liang Jiang & Xiang Fu
One warms, the other moves
Together they effectively
warm the Stomach, drain Cold,
move the Qi and stop pain
> *Liang Fu Wan* (only these 2 herbs in formula)

Ma Huang & Yin Xing (Bai Guo)
Ma Huang unblocks and redirects Lung Qi, and releases the Exterior.
Yin Xing transforms Phlegm and contains the leakage of Lung Qi.
Additionally, Yin Xing prevents Ma Huang
from causing excessive dispersion and depletion.
Both herbs arrest wheezing.
Together their complementary actions of dispersing and binding
Greatly enhances the ability of *Ding Chuan Tang* to **arrest wheezing.**
> *Ding Chuan Tang*

Chen Pi & Zhu Ru
One is Warm, the other is Cold
Together they clear and warm simultaneously
Eliminating mixed Cold and Heat in the Stomach
They harmonize the Stomach,
Descend rebellious Qi and stop vomiting
> *Ju Pi Zhu Ru Tang*
> (note: *Ju Pi* is the recent skin, whereas *Chen Pi* is the aged skin)

Formulas
Regulate Qi

Yue Ju Wan
Ban Xia Hou Po Tang
Gua Lou Xie Bai Bai Jiu Tang
Gua Lou Xie Bai Ban Xia Tang
Zhi Shi Gua Lou Gui Zhi Tang
Liang Fu Wan

Tian Tai Wu Yao San
Su Zi Jiang Qi Tang
Ding Chuan Tang
Xuan Fu Dai Zhe Tang
Ju Pi Zhu Ru Tang

Promote Movement of Qi

1. Plum-pit qi (*mei he qi*) resulting from emotional upset due to circumstances which are figuratively hard to swallow:

2. Stagnation of Liver Qi with Cold Congealing in the Stomach:

3. For focal distension, this formula is frequently used in treating mild cases of constraint due to stagnant qi: Yue Ju Wan (disturbance of qi, blood & fire associated with Liver, which affects middle jiao, then causing damp phlegm, and food stagnation)

4. Painful obstruction of the chest from Yang deficiency affecting the Upper Jiao (main formula):

5. In cases where the chest pain is so severe the patient cannot lie down, more severe phlegm accumulation, add (herb):
Formula:

6. Painful obstruction of chest with fullness and pain, or a stabbing pain radiating from chest to back. This formula is more effective (than the principle formula) of severe clumping of qi resulting in focal distention in the chest:

7. Lower abdominal pain radiating to the testicles due to stagnation in the Liver channel due to Cold:

Direct Rebellious Qi Downward
8. Wheezing caused by Exterior Wind Cold and Phlegm Heat smoldering in the Interior:

9. Phlegm turbidity obstructing the Interior with Stomach Qi deficiency:

10. Excess Phlegm Cold in the Lungs above, and deficient Kidney Qi below:

11. Stomach Heat and either rebellious Stomach Qi or injured Stomach Qi (from severe diarrhea or vomiting):

Yue Ju Wan	Ban Xia Hou Po Tang	Ju Pi Zhu Ru Tang
1. Damp:	Two title herbs:	Two title herbs:
2. Blood:	1.	1.
3. Qi:	2.	2.
4. Heat:	Leach out Dampness:	Tonify Qi (with *Chen Pi* regulates):
5. Food:	3.	3.
	Harmonize, stop vomiting:	Three amigos (*sheng g.c.*)
	4.	4.
	Light, warm, Lung ch:	5.
	5.	6.

Invigorate Blood

Tao He Cheng Qi Tang
Xue Fu Zhu Yu Tang
Tong Qiao Huo Xue Tang
Ge Xia Zhu Yu Tang
Shao Fu Zhu Yu Tang
Shen Tong Zhu Yu Tang

Shi Xiao San
Da Huang Zhe Chong Wan
Gui Zhi Fu Ling Wan
Sheng Hua Tang
Wen Jing Tang

Zhu Yu Tang: drive out blood stasis
Xue Fu: Blood Mansion
Ge Xia: below the diaphragm
Shao Fu: lower abdomen ("lesser abdomen)
Tong Qiao: unblock the orifices (of the head)

Invigorate Blood & Dispel Stasis
1. Blood Stasis in the Head, face or upper body:

2. Blood buildup in the Lower Burner caused by the accumulation of Blood Stasis and Heat:

3. Blood stasis in the chest with impairment of blood flow in the area above the diaphragm (complicated by constrained Liver Qi):

4. Blood stasis accumulating in the lower abdomen (with masses or pain):

5. Blood Stasis and Liver Qi stagnation below the diaphragm with palpable abdominal masses:

6. Painful obstruction due to the obstruction of Qi and Blood in the channels:

7. Retention of Blood stasis that obstructs the vessels of the lower abdomen causing irregular menses and dysmenorrhea (post child birth):

8. Accumulation of dry blood (from consumption, chronic debilitating disorders, extreme weakness, and deficient yuan qi):

Warm the Menses & Dispel Blood Stasis
9. Post-Partum Cold with Qi & Blood deficiency:

10. Deficiency and Cold of the Ren and Chong, with Blood Stasis obstruction:

11. Blood stasis in the womb (restless fetus, bleeding during pregnancy):

WEEK 9

Influential Points
Zang:
Fu:
Sinews:
Marrow:
Qi:
Bones:
Blood:
Vessels:

Chrono-Acupuncture
(2 hour segments of dominant zang fu organs)

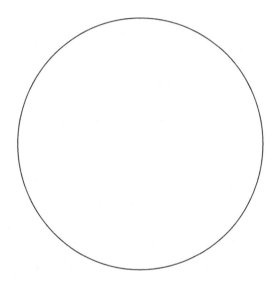

1. If you treat an organ during the 2 hour period *after* the organ time or opposite, is it tonification or sedation?
2. If you treat an organ during the 2 hour period of the organ, is it tonification or sedation?
3. So which two time periods could you tonify the Stomach? 9-11am (Spleen time) or 7-9pm (Pericardium time)
4. 11pm-1am:
The qi is _____ during its time period, and _____ at the opposite side of the clock.
5. Therefore when the Qi of the Stomach is strongest when?
6. And when the Qi of the Heart is the strongest which channel is the weakest?

Meridian Theory & Points Review Questions:

1. Facial paralysis: (list 1 distal point and 2 local points):
2. Uterine bleeding, direct moxa (list 2 possible points):
3. Night sweats:
4. Spleen point to treat Dampness:
5. Stomach point to treat Phlegm/Dampness:
6. Stomach point for shoulder pain:
7. GB point for shoulder pain (or pain/motor impairment of any joint):
8. Liv point for clearing Fire:
9. Stomach point for clearing Fire/Heat:
10. Sudden loss of voice & stiff tongue (probably post-stroke):
11. Lung Heat/Fire:
12. Lung Def:
13. Lung point for hemoptysis:
14. To turn a breech baby, direct moxa on which point:
15. SI point to treat acute pain of neck or low back:
16. SI point for shoulder & vision problems:
17. What other type of point is the luo point often combined with?
18. Which luo point is the command point for the head and neck?
19. Which He Sea point specifically treats summer heat and low back pain?
20. Which luo point is the confluent point of the Chong?
21. Which luo point on the leg treats blurring vision, opthalmalgia, night blindness and distending pain of the breast?
22. List 5 causes of blood stasis:
23. Use the front mu points to treat zang or fu?
24. Back shu to treat zang or fu?
25. Which front mu point is located below the nipple in the 7th intercostals space?
26. Which front mu is indicated for chest pain and fullness, asthma, palpitation, insufficient lactation, hiccup and difficulty swallowing?
27. Influential point of zang is located where?
28. Front mu of the _____ is also the influential point of fu organs
29. Influential point of qi is located level with Spleen _____
30. Influential point of vessels is located over which artery?
31. Influential point of bone is located level with which vertebra?]
32. What point is also located at the same level Du 13, UB 11,
33. Influential point of marrow is located _____ cun above the lateral malleolus
33. Influential point of tendons is _____ and located _____ & _____ to the head of which bone_____
34. Which go from the extremities to the head and trunk and do not go to the zang fu?
    a. Luo
    b. Divergent
    c. Muscle Tendon

Fill in (Jing Well, Ying Spring, Shu Stream, Jing River, He Sea)
37. _____ are for painful joints
38. _____ are for disease of Stomach and Intestines
39. _____ emergency resuscitation & cardiac pain
40. _____ asthma
41. _____ fever

42. Ear problems can be treated with which 3 of the 12 regular channels?
43. Mental symptoms may be seen on which 3 Regular Channels:
44. Which of the eight extra channels connect with the eyes?

45. Which regular channels connect with the eyes:
46. Which channel connects with both the inner and outer canthus?
47. Which points to treat insufficient lactation and mastitis? (list 4)
48. For hypochondriac pain due to blood stasis, and famous for constipation:
49. Points associates with throat, chest, and lungs (8 extra pairs):
    a. SI 3, UB 62
    b. Lu 7, K 6
    c. GB 41, SJ 5
    d. P 6, Sp 4

50. Sudden onset or bleeding disorders choose points from what category?
51. Which one is *not* a muscle tendon channel symptoms:
    a. swelling,
    b. pain,
    c. spasm,
    d. redness
52. Foot yin muscle tendon channels converge at:
53. Hand yin muscle tendon channels converge at:
54. Foot Yang muscle tendon channels converge at:
55. Hand Yang channels converge:
56. For Zang organ dz choose points from which two categories?
57. For Fu organ dz choose points from which two categories?
58. For cardiac pain, nausea and vomiting, choose points from which channel?
59. Water metabolism problems with ear problems, use which channel?
60. Which channels do *not* have independent symptoms (separate from the associated regular channel):
    a. divergent
    b. muscle tendon
    c. 8 extra
    d. 12 regular

Order of qi flow in the channels:
1. Hand Tai Yin, Lung
2.
3.
4.
5.
6.
7.
8.
9.
10
11.
12.

Zang Fu Syndrome Review Questions (cases)

1. Sx: feeble cough, clear & dilute phlegm, spontaneous sweating, shortness of breath worse on exertion, lack of desire to talk.
T: pale, thin white fur   P: weak & def
Dx:

2. Sx: burning hypochondriac pain, dizziness, vertigo, tinnitus, red eyes, irritable, hematemesis, hemoptysis, epistaxis, yellow urine & constipation
T: red body, yellow coat   P: bowstring rapid
Dx:

3. Sx: pale complexion, poor appetite, loose stool, distended abdomen worse after eating, dull abdominal pain better with warmth and pressure, cold limbs
T: pale, white coat   P: deep, slow (could be weak also)
Dx:

4. Sx: loss of appetite, abdominal fullness & distension, loose stool or diarrhea, heaviness of the head & body, sticky saliva
T: white, sticky coat   P: soft
Dx:

5. Sx: palpitations, insomnia, dream disturbed sleep, poor memory, pale complexion, dizziness, verrtigo
T: pale   P: thready, weak
Dx:

6. Sx: palpitations, insomnia, dream disturbed sleep, poor memory, tidal fever, night sweats
T: red, less fur   P: thready rapid
Dx: Heart Yin Def

7. Sx: enuresis, incontinence, premature ejaculation
Dx:

8. Sx: dizziness, vertigo, tinnitus, distending headache, red eyes, irritable, insomnia, dream disturbed sleep, palpitations, poor memory, sore low back & knees
T: red   P: bowstring, thready, rapid
Dx:

9. Sx: irritable & depressed, breast distension, stuffy chest, sighing, abdominal distension & pain, poor appetite, belching
T: thin white coat   P: bowstring
Dx:

10. Sx: profuse white sputum, shortness of breath, fullness/stuffiness in chest
T: white sticky coat   P: slippery
Dx:

11. Sx: insomnia, flushed face, mouth ulcers, thirst, deep yellow painful urination
T: red   P: rapid
Dx:

12. Sx: cough, possible fever and chills, absence of sweating, headache, nasal discharge
T: thin white coat   P: floating tight
Dx:

13. Sx: dizziness & tinnitus, insomnia, poor memory, nocturnal emission, afternoon fever, malar flush, night sweating, yellow urine & constipation, sore low back & knees

T: red, less coat   P: thready, rapid

Dx:

HERBS

TONIFY YANG

herb (yao 藥)	flavor (wei 味)		temp (qi 氣)	channels					
lu rong	**sweet**, salty		**warm**	K	Liv				(Du)
ge jie	salty		neutral	K		Lu			
dong chong xia cao	**swet**		**warm**	K		Lu			
rou cong rong	**sweet**, salty		**warm**	K			LI		
suo yang	**sweet**		**warm**	K	Liv		LI		
yin yang huo	acrid, **sweet**		**warm**	K	Liv				
ba ji tian	acrid, **sweet**		**warm**	K	Liv				
hu lu ba	bitter		**warm**	K	Liv				
hu tao ren	**sweet**		**warm**	K		Lu	LI		
bu gu zhi	acrid, bitter		**very warm**	K				Sp	
yi zhi ren	acrid		**warm**	K				Sp	
xian mao	acrid	toxic	**hot**	K	Liv				
du zhong	**sweet**, sl. acrid		warm	K	Liv				
gou ji	bitter, **sweet**		warm	K	Liv				
xu duan	bitter, acrid		sl. warm	K	Liv				
gu sui bu	bitter		**warm**	K	Liv				
tu si zi	acrid, **sweet**		neutral	K	Liv				
sha yuan ji li	**sweet**		**warm**	K	Liv				
zi he che	**sweet**, salty		warm	K	Liv	Lu			

TONIFY BLOOD

herb (yao 藥)	flavor (wei 味)		temp (qi 氣)	channels				
shu di huang	**sweet**		**sl. warm**	Ht	K	Liv		
he shou wu	**bitter, sweet**	astringent	**sl. warm**		K	Liv		
dang gui	sweet, acrid, bitter		**warm**	Ht		Liv	Sp	
bai shao	bitter, sour		cool			Liv	Sp	
e jiao	sweet		neutral		K	Liv		Lu
gou qi zi	sweet		**neutral**		K	Liv	Lu	
sang shen	sweet		**cold**	Ht	K	Liv		
long yan rou	**sweet**		**warm**	Ht				

Herbs
Tonify Yang

Lu Rong	**Yin Yang Huo (Xian Ling Pi)**	**Yi Zhi Ren**
Ge Jie	*Ba Ji Tian*	*Xian Mao*
Dong Chong Xia Cao	*Hu Lu Ba*	*Du Zhong*
Rou Cong Rong	*Hu Tao Ren*	*Gou Ji*
Suo Yang	*Bu Gu Zhi*	*Xu Duan*
Gu Sui Bu	**Tu Si Zi**	**Sha Yuan Ji Li**
Zi He Che		

Rou Cong Rong & Suo Yang both tonify Kidney Yang and moisten the Intestines.

1. _____ *is regarded as the more moistening, while*

2. _____ *more powerfully tonifies Yang.*

Bai Ji Tian, Yin Yang Huo & Xian Mao *all tonify Kidney Yang, strengthen the sinews and expel Wind Damp.*

3. _____ *is the strongest, and toxic, so although it is very effective it should not be taken long term.*

4. _____ *is extremely drying (which can injure the yin) but it is particularly effective for Kidney Yang deficient Bi syndrome.*

5. _____ *is relatively mild, not very drying, augments the essence and strengthens sinews and bones (good for Damp Cold Yang Deficiency).*

Du Zhong, Xu Duan, Gou Ji & Sang Ji Sheng all tonify the Liver & Kidneys and strengthen the Bones and Tendons.

6. _____ is the warmest, and is stronger at expelling Wind Damp Cold. Used for chronic Bi syndrome.

7. _____ is bitter, sweet and neutral and is the weakest for tonifying the Liver and Kidney and strengthening Bones and tendons, but it can tonify the Blood and expel Wind Damp.

8. _____ has the strongest tonifying action, and gently regulates Qi & Blood.

9. _____ is similar to the herb in question 8, but weaker in tonifying the Kidney, and perhaps more effective in strengthening the bones and tendons (as its name 'connect broken' implies).

10. Three of the four herbs in the above question can prevent miscarriage or calm a restless fetus:
_____ , _____ , & _____ .

11. Sweet, salty & warm, _____ tonifies the Du, stabilizes the Ren & Chong and is probably the strongest Yang tonic for the Liver and Kidney. It augments the essence & Blood and strengthens Sinews and Bones.

12. Acrid, bitter and very warm, _____ is also astringent, and therefore and important herb for Spleen and Kidney Yang deficiency.

13. In addition to tonifying the Kidney, _____ promotes Blood movement for trauma, taken internally or applied topically (as a tincture topically for alopecia).

The following two herbs both benefit the vision.

14. _____ evenly tonifies Kidney Yin and Yang, and also binds Essence. It improves vision, warms the Spleen to stop Diarrhea, and stabilizes the Ren & Chong to calm the fetus.

15. _____ mildly tonifies the Liver and Kidney and improves visual acuity.

16. _____ warms and tonifies, stabilizes and bind (for diarrhea, frequent urination and spermatorrhea).

17. _____ tonifies Yin, Yang, Qi and Blood, and so may treat all patterns of deficiency, including insufficient lactation. Also tonifies the Lung Qi for wheezing.

18. _____ benefits the Kidneys and tonifies the Lungs and is very good for wheezing (the head and feet are usually not used in decoctions)

19. Tonifies Kidney Yang and Lung Yin, and therefore because of its balanced nature can be taken long term. It is sweet, warm, and enters the Lung and Kidney, and is endangered in its high plateau native environment due to over-harvesting.

Nourish Blood

Shu Di Huang	*E Jiao*
He Shou Wu	*Gou Qi Zi*
Dang Gui	*Sang Shen*
Bai Shao	*Long Yan Rou*

1. In its raw form _____ is used for moistening the Intestine. Prepared form to tonify the Liver and Kidneys, nourish the Blood and augment the essence, famous for prematurely graying hair.

2. _____ is the Imperial herb for tonifying and invigorating the Blood and for regulating menses and alleviating pain. The head is more tonifying and the tail more invigorating.

3. _____ is sweet, warm and cloying and nourishes Yin and Blood, replenishes essence and augments the marrow. Primarily used for essence and Blood deficiency. Often combined with Sha Ren to counteract its cloying nature.

4. _____ nourishes the Liver Blood, augments the Kidney Yin, moistens the Lung and stops bleeding (often used for bleeding due to Blood Deficiency)

5. Sweet and warm, and entering the Heart and Spleen, _____ calms the spirit for insomnia due to Heart and Spleen Deficiency.

6. _____ tonifies the Kidney to augment Essence and Blood, and nourishes the Liver to enhance visual acuity (one of the richest sources of betacarotene good for night vision)

7. Nourishes Yin and Blood, generates fluid, and moistens the Intestines. (Used in syrup form)

8. Sour and bitter, _____ enters the Liver channel to nourish Liver Blood and protect Liver Yin, calm and descend Liver Yang and clear Liver Fire. (Also enters the Spleen channel)

<u>*Fang Feng & Huang Qi*</u>
One dissipates and opens
The other supplements and secures
***Huang Qi* supplements the *Wei Qi* without retaining pathogens**
Fang Feng* drains pathogens without damaging the *ZhengQi
Together they effectively secure the exterior and supplement the *Wei Qi*
Dispel and prevent further invasion by pathogens, and stop sweating
    Yu Ping Feng San

<u>Bu Gu Zhi & Rou Dou Kou</u>
One is warming and supplements the Kidneys
The other is astringing and supplements the Spleen
Together they effectively supplement Spleen & Kidney Yang,
Secure the Intestines and stop daybreak diarrhea
    Si Shen Wan

<u>Formulas: *Stop Bleeding*</u>

Shi Hui San
Si Sheng Wan
Jiao Ai Tang

Clear Heat & Stop Bleeding
1. Upper burner manifestations of Blood Heat:

2. Fire blazing in the middle and upper burners, injures the vessels and causes reckless blood (associated with Liver Fire attacking the Stomach):

Tonify & Stop Bleeding
3. Injury and Deficiency of the Ren and Chong:

Yu Ping Feng San
Zhen Ren Yang Zang Tang
Tao Hua Tang
Si Shen Wan
Jin Suo Gu Jing Wan

Sang Piao Xiao San
Suo Quan Wan
Gu Jing Wan
Wan Dai Tang

Stabilize the Exterior & Lungs
1. Deficient *Wei Qi*:

Restrain Intestine Leakage
2. Kidney (& Spleen) Yang Deficient 'daybreak diarrhea':

3. Middle Jiao (and Kidney) Yang Deficiency (although initially dysentery is usually Damp Heat, after it damages the Middle Jiao turns into Yang Deficient Cold):

4. Fluid loss from chronic diarrhea, with Spleen Qi deficiency and Intestines unable to absorb:

Stabilize the Kidneys
5. Kidney & Liver Yin deficiency (or K essence def) causing spermatorrhea:

6. Kidney & Heart Qi Deficiency causing frequent cloudy urination & possible spermatorrhea:

7. Kidney Qi Deficiency, failing to transform Bladder Qi (Deficient Cold):

Stabilize the Womb
8. Dai dysfunction causing leukorrhea (with Spleen Qi Deficiency and Liver Qi impaired, further weakening the Spleen):

9. Liver Qi stagnation causing Heat which disturbs the Ren & Chong causing Hot reckless Blood (continuous menstruation or uterine bleeding):

Yu Ping Feng San vs. *Gui Zhi Tang*
Both for treating Exterior Deficiency Conditions
Gui Zhi Tang: relatively acute conditions with fever & aversion to cold,
     Where sweating does not resolve the problem, *Xie Qi* is strong
Yu Ping Feng San: chronic problems marked by spontaneous sweating
     With aversion to drafts and recurrent colds, *Zheng Qi* Deficiency

Case Studies of Formulas that Stabilize & Bind

1. Continuous menstruation or uterine bleeding that alternates between trickling and gushing of blood. The blood is very red and may contain dark purple clots. Accompanying signs and symptoms include a sensation of Heat and irritability in the chest, abdominal pain, dark urine
T: red
P: rapid, wiry
Fx:

2. Chronic spermatorrhea, impotence, fatigue and weakness, sore and weak limbs, lower back pain, tinnitus
T: pale with white coat
P: thin, frail
Fx:

3. Profuse vaginal discharge that is white or pale yellow in color, thin consistency, no particular smell, usually continuous, also fatigue, lethargy, shiny pale complexion, loose stool
T: pale with white coat
P: soggy and frail or moderate
Fx:

4. Daybreak diarrhea, no interest in food, poor digestion, sore low back, cold limbs, fatigue, lethargy, possible abdominal pain
T: pale with thin white coat
P: submerged slow and forceless
Fx:

5. Chronic diarrhea or dysentery
Two formulas:
1.
2.

6. Aversion to drafts, spontaneous sweating, recurrent colds, shiny pale complexion
T: pale with white coat
P: floating, deficient and soft
Fx:

7. Frequent clear and prolonged urination or enuresis
T: pale with white coat
P: submerged frail (deep weak)
Fx:

8. Frequent urination (possibly incontinent), urine the color of rice water (grey & cloudy), possible spermatorrhea, disorientation, forgetfulness
T: pale with white coat
P: thin, slow, frail
Fx:

WEEK 10
Needling & Treatment Techniques

_Bu_ (Reinforcing), _Xie_ (Reducing) & Even Technique

1. Open hole:
2. Closed hole:

3. Four Animal Techniques (dragon, tiger, turtle, phoenix) are used for:
   a. Opening the channels & moving Qi
   b. Tonifying Qi
   c. Reducing Xie Qi

The following techniques are used for (you should know the method of treatment too):

   4. Green Dragon Wags its Tail:

   5. White Tiger Shakes its head

   6. Black Turtle Searches the Hole

   7. Red Phoenix Meets the Source

   8. Dragon & Tiger Fighting (for pain relief)

   9. Guiding Qi (Dao Qi) Technique

   10. Yin Hidden in Yang:

   11. Yang Hidden in Yin:

   12. Setting the Moutnain on Fire (3 levels down):

   13. Sky Cooling (3 levels up):

Bleeding (3 edge needle)
4. Function:
5. bleed UB 40 for:
6. bleed Lu 11 for:
7. bleed the ear apex for:
8. Bleeding is contraindicated for:

Contraindications for needling:
9. Pregnant women 1st trimester
10. Pregnant women 2nd & 3rd trimester:
11. Infants:

12. If a patient faints, what do you do first:

14. Gua Sha is best for treating diseases in which part of the body: (deep or exterior)

15. 7 Star Needling is used to treat what types of diseases:

Moxa
16. Functions:
17. with ginger:
18. with garlic:
19. with Fu Zi:
20. Contraindications:

week 10

Selected Points for Common Symtpoms
(from Shanghai, p. 556-557)

Fever:

Fainting:

Shock, moxa:

Shock needle:

Spontaneous sweating:

Night Sweating:

Insomnia:

Aphasia (stiff tongue/tongue paralysis):

Palpitations:

Chest Pain:

Cough:

Nausea & vomiting:

Hypochondriac Pain:

Constipation:

Pruritis (itching):

Herbs
Tonify Yin

(Bei) Sha Shen	Yu Zhu	Hei Zhi Ma
Xi Yang Shen	Bai He	Gui Ban
Tian Men Dong	(Sang Ji Sheng)	Bie Jia
Mai Men Dong	Han Lian Cao	(Luo Han Guo)
Shi Hu	Nu Zhen Zi	

Both: Sweet & Sour generate Yin
        Sweet & Cold generate Yin

1. Sang Shen & Gou Qi Zi are moistening and the tonify both _____ & _____.

Main Men Dong & Tian Men Dong both nourish Yin & moisten dryness. They are combined for mutual reinforcemnt for Lung dryness with cough.

2. _____ is extremely cold, strongly clears Heat & moistens Dryness. It enters the Kidney channel to nourish Kidney Yin.

3. _____ enters the Heart channel to clear Heart heat and eliminate irritability. Also enters the Stomach channel to generate fluid.

4. _____ mildly and evenly tonifies the Liver and Kidneys.

Sha Shen, Shi Hu & Yu Zhu are often combined for mutual reinforcement for Lung & St Yin Def.

5. _____ enhances visual acuity and focuses on nourishing Stomach Yin.

6. _____ tonifies without retaining pathogenic factors. It is used in cooking sometimes.

7. _____ is effective in nourishing Lung Yin.

8. Sweet, slightly bitter and cold, _____ tonifeis the Qi and nourishes Yin. It enters the Heart, Lung & Kidneys.

9. _____ mostiens the Lung and clears Heart heat, often used for dyr cough and also for irritability and insomnia. (It is the *Jun* herb of a formula for Lung Dryness due to Lung & Kidney Yin Deficiency causing cough with blood streaked sputum)

10. Contraindicated during pregnancy, _____ acts on the Ren and greatly tonifies Kidney Yin and anchors Yang. Additionally it benefitst he Kidney and strengthens bones (often combined with Lu Rong).

12. Salty and cold, _____ nourishes Yin, anchors Yang and more strongly clears Heat. Additionally it invigorates Blood, softens hardness, dissipates nodules and is contraindicated in pregnancy.

13. Bonus herb (do not need to know for comps) _____ is good for pregnant women to treat thirst and dry throat instead of *Tian Hua Fen* (which is C/I in pregnancy). It is sweet and neutral, and moistens and cools the Lung.

Astringent

Shan Zhu Yu	Shi Liu Pi	Bai Guo
Wu Wei Zi	Lian Zi	Fu Xiao Mai
Wu Mei	Qian Shi	Ma Huang Gen
He Zi	Jin Ying Zi	Hai Piao Xiao
Rou Dou Kou	Fu Pen Zi	Sang Piao Xiao
Ying Su Ke	Wu Bei Zi	

Fu Xiao Mai & Ma Huang Gen both stop abnormal swating and treat spontaneous & night sweating. They are commonly used for mutual reinforcemnt.

1. _____ is astringent and exclusively restrains abnormal sweat.

2. _____ is sweet and cold to augment Qi, eliminate heat and stop abnormal sweating (it is in a 3-herb formula for restless organ disorder)

Qian Shi & Lian Zi both strengthen the Spleen and stop diarrhea, augment the Kidney and bind the essence (*jing*). They also are commonly combined for mutual reinforcement.

3. _____ is stronger at strengthening the Splena dn stopping diarrhea, also enters the Heart channel to nourish the Heart and calm the *Shen* (to treat the heart, better to have the 'heart' center of the herb still inside)

4. _____ is stronger in augmenting the Kidney and binding essence (*jing*).

Sang Piao Xiao & Hai Piao Xiao both augment the Kidney and bind the essence

5. _____ assists the Kidney Yang to restrain and bind the essence (*jing*). It astringes while tonifying.

6. _____ exclusively restrains without having any tonifying effects. It astringes to stop bleeding, and also reduces acidity, alleviates pain, resolves dampness and promotes the healing of sores.

Shan Zhu Yu & Wu Wei Zi are strong astringents and have a wide variety of applications including some tonifying action.

7. _____ focuses on the Liver, Kidneys & essence (*jing*), and (important part of *Liu Wei Di Huang Wan*)

8. _____ focuses more on the Lugns and Kindeys, specifically the Kidney's ability to grasp the Qi to support healthy breathing (important part of a 3-herb formula for tonifying Lung Yin & Qi, generate fluids and stop excessive sweating)

Wu Mei & He Zi work on both the Lungs and the Large Intestine.

9. _____ has a stronger descending actiona dn can be used for treating phlegm-heat affecting the throat and Lugns

10. _____ generates fluids and can also e used against intestinal parasites

11. The wheezing arresting action of _____ is so strong it is used for excess conditions as well as deficiency. 21 pieces are prescribed as the *Jun* herb in a formula to arrest wheezing due to phlegm-heat int eh Lungs.

12. A naturally rich source of vitamin C, _____ stabilizes the Kidney sfor all kinds of lower jiao leakage (spermatorrhea, urinary incontinence and vaginal discharge) and binds the intestines.

13. _____ enters the Kidney & Liver, and besides augmenting and stabilizing the Kidny, it has a specific function of improving vision.

14. _____ contains the leakage of Lung Qi, binds the Intestines for chronic diarrhea and is famous world-wide for its ability to alleviate any kind of pain (not for this last function in Chinese medicine, and actually not used clinically in the U.S.)

15. _____ acts on the Intestines to stop diarrhea and the middle jiao to warm, move Qi and alleviate pain (featured as one of the four miracles *Si Shen* that stops diarrhea).

16. A less frequently used herb, _____ is sour, astringent, warm and toxic. It binds the intestines, stabilizes the Kidny and retains essence and kills parasites (internally for tapeworms and roundworms, topically for ringworm)

17. Sour, salty and cold, _____ contains the leakage of Lung Qi, preserves and restrains (for spermatorrhea, sweating, or bleeding), and absorbs moisture to reduce hot toxic swelling. It is used topically to treat scar tissue.

Formulas: *Calm Spirit*

Tian Wang Bu Xin Dan　　　*Gan Mai Da Zao Tang*
Suan Zao Ren Tang　　　　*Zhu Sha An Shen Wan*

Nourish the Heart & Calm Spirit
1. Liver & Heart Blood Deficiency with Deficient Heat:

2. Yin Deficiency of the Heart and Kidneys (with deficient Heat):

3. Restless Organ Disorder (*Zang Zao*), attributed to excessive worry, anxiety or pensiveness which injures Heart Yin, disrupts Liver Qi flow and affects Spleen Qi:

Sedate & Calm Spirit
4. Vigorous Heart Fire injuring the Blood and Yin:

Expel Wind

Xiao Feng San　　　　　*Tian Ma Gou Teng*
Xiao Huo Luo Dan　　　*E Jiao Yi Zi Huang Tang*
Qian Zheng San　　　　　YinDi Huang Yin Zi

Release Wind from the Skin & Channels
1. After the onset of Wind Stroke, Dampness, Phlegm and lifeless Blood obstruct the channels and collaterals:

2. Wind Heat or Wind Damp invading with pre-existing Damp Heat (which settles in the Blood) transforming into Wind Toxin:

3. Sequelae of channel stroke with symptoms confined th the head and face (facial paralysis, including due to Bell's Palsey):

Extinguish Internal Wind
4. Internal Wind from Blood and Yin Def:

5. Ascendant Liver Yang with Internal Liver Wind:

6. Mute Paraplegia due to Kidney Yin and Yang Deficiency with Deficient Fire:

Open Orifices

An Gong Niu Huang Wan　　*Zi Xue Dan*
Zhi Bao Dan　　　　　　*Su He Xiang Wan*

Clear Heat & Open the Orifices
1. Blazing Heat sinking into the Pericardium generating Internal Liver Wind:

2. Warm febrile disease sinking into the Pericardium with turbid phlegm veiling the sensory orifices (also for Closed type Wind Stroke, focuses on clearing Heat and relieving toxicity, most cooling of these formulas):

3. Heat sinking into the Pericardium creating confusion by disturbing the Spirit (focuses on clearing phlegm and aromatically opening the orifices, least cooling of these formulas)

Warm & Open the Orifices
4. Cold Damp and turbid phlegm veiling the sensory orifices:

Made in the USA
Las Vegas, NV
21 December 2023

83433024R00077